Becoming a Mental Health Counselor

A Guide to Career Development and Professional Identity

■ ■ ■

Adam M. Volungis
Assumption University

ROWMAN & LITTLEFIELD
Lanham • Boulder • New York • London

Acquisitions Editor: Mark Kerr
Acquisitions Assistant: Courtney Packard
Sales and Marketing Inquiries: textbooks@rowman.com

Credits and acknowledgments for material borrowed from other sources, and reproduced with permission, appear on the appropriate pages within the text.

Published by Rowman & Littlefield
An imprint of The Rowman & Littlefield Publishing Group, Inc.
4501 Forbes Boulevard, Suite 200, Lanham, Maryland 20706
www.rowman.com

6 Tinworth Street, London SE11 5AL, United Kingdom

British Library Cataloguing in Publication Information Available

Library of Congress Cataloging-in-Publication Data
Names: Volungis, Adam M., author.
Title: Becoming a mental health counselor : a guide to career development and professional
    identity / Adam M. Volungis, Assumption University.
Description: Lanham : Rowman & Littlefield, [2022] | Includes bibliographical references
    and index.
Identifiers: LCCN 2021018202 (print) | LCCN 2021018203 (ebook) | ISBN 9781538121160
    (cloth) | ISBN 9781538121177 (paperback) | ISBN 9781538121184 (epub)
Subjects: LCSH: Mental health counselors—Vocational guidance. | Mental health
    counseling—Vocational guidance.
Classification: LCC RC466 .V65 2022 (print) | LCC RC466 (ebook) | DDC 362.2023—dc23
LC record available at https://lccn.loc.gov/2021018202
LC ebook record available at https://lccn.loc.gov/2021018203

Dedication
To Yeonjoo and Kai: My inspirations to keep moving forward
To My Parents: Thank you for your unconditional love
and support

Contents

■ ■ ■

Detailed Contents

■ ■ ■

Preface

■ ■ ■

I am a counseling psychologist and have been a licensed mental health counselor for over 15 years. For the past six years, I have taught a course called "Issues in Professional Practice" in our clinical counseling psychology program, which introduces our students to the varied facets of professional practice and development in counseling. Topics covered range from obtaining licensure and a high-quality job to self-care and professional identity. While teaching this course, I soon realized that something was missing. Although there are a few great books tailored to the applied practice of mental health counselors, there is not much out there that focuses solely on career development and professional growth (e.g., self-care and preventing burnout, the licensure application process, how to apply for a job in the mental health field). It is important to note that this text is not aligned with any one professional association (American Counseling Association or American Mental Health Counselors Association), accreditation board (Council for Accreditation of Counseling and Related Education Programs or Masters in Psychology and Counseling Accreditation Council), or type of graduate degree (counselor education or clinical counseling psychology). The goal of this book is to be an inclusive primary source of professional career basics for mental health counselors of all different training backgrounds.

The following highlights the key themes for each of the eight chapters in this book:

Chapter 1 focuses on assessing if being a mental health counselor is the right career choice for you. Whether you are confident in your career choice to enter the mental health field or you have some ambiguous thoughts and feelings, this chapter will hopefully at least get you thinking about your key qualities and personal motivation for pursuing a career in counseling. Self-awareness and coping with personal issues, multicultural awareness and sensitivity, and the importance of evidence-based practice also is addressed. Mental health counseling can be a demanding profession, but it also has its rewards!

Chapter 2 provides a relatively brief review of professional identity development and professional ethics. The focus of this chapter is to highlight the most relevant points within the scope of preparing you to be a professional mental health counselor. Professional identity development includes consideration of such components as education and accreditation, scope and approach to practice, specialization (including population served and setting), and intrapersonal and interpersonal dimensions. Professional ethics focuses on the necessity for having an established code of ethics, ethical decision-making, legal and ethical issues in counseling, and strategies to ensure ethical practice, including reviewing ethical codes of special interest to mental health counselors and proactive approaches to avoid conflicts with specific codes.

Chapter 3 focuses on education and licensure requirements to be a mental health counselor. It takes much time, commitment, and money from entering graduate school to getting licensed. The last thing you want is the added stress of scrambling toward the end of your journey, making sure that you can get licensed. Although there are variations across all 50 states, there are also many core similarities. One obvious and major first step is getting the appropriate graduate degree in counseling, including program qualities, curriculum, accreditation, and practicum and internship training opportunities. Thereafter, there are important postgraduate experiences such as getting the appropriate number of supervised counseling hours and obtaining quality supervision. You will also need to consider certification and licensure exam requirements, including a detailed focus on the two most common licensure exams: National Counselor Examination and National Clinical Mental Health Counseling Examination. Finally, there is the licensure application itself. It is important to prepare for all the requirements and follow all the instructions to expedite application time and reduce distress. It is a long journey from graduating with your degree in counseling to obtaining the required counseling hours postgraduation. However, the journey is well worth it and quite an accomplishment!

Chapter 4 reviews expectations for mental health counselors beyond counseling. To be a successful counselor, you will need many skills beyond what happens in the counseling room with your clients. In other words, you will need good communication and writing skills. The expectations beyond counseling addressed in this chapter include paperwork (e.g., intake assessment, case formulation and treatment plan, progress note, and discharge plan and summary), case management, working with colleagues, supervision, managed care organizations, and professional advocacy. Mental health counselors have many responsibilities in addition to counseling clients.

Chapter 5 discusses some of the unique details of applying for and obtaining a job as a mental health counselor. Although there are certainly overlaps in many of the steps to searching for a job in general, there are also some nuances in the mental health field that need to be taken into consideration. Looking for a job is a lot like dating. You want to make sure that there is a good match for both you and your future employer. Searching for a desirable job includes starting early with at least some focus on a preferred population to work with and a setting to work in. You should also consider available benefits beyond salary. The job search itself includes not only online skills but also networking skills. Much effort should be put into developing your résumé and cover letter. This is often what is first seen by potential employers and is a key factor in determining whether you get invited for an interview. Before any face-to-face interviews, you will probably be interviewed online, without you even knowing it. More and more potential employers are using the Internet to screen candidates before offering an interview. Because of this, there are key strategies that should be followed to manage your online reputation. The last thing you want to have happen is to not get offered an interview because something less than flattering about you is available online for all to see. Of course, the actual face-to-face interview is vital to potential employment. Important factors to consider are research and practice before your interview, how you present yourself, how you communicate (verbal and nonverbal), and how you answer questions and ask questions. Finally, after your interview, there are still more parts of the process to consider: processing your interview experience, saying "thank you," following up, responding to offers, and responding to rejections. Job hunting is both a science and an art. The more time and effort you put into the process, the greater your chances for obtaining a job that matches your interests and values.

Chapter 6 addresses the growing concern of burnout in mental health counselors. Because counseling by nature is a one-way caring relationship, where clients express intense emotions and share difficult life events, it is not surprising that many counselors experience physical and emotional exhaustion. Burnout is a concern for not only your own mental health well-being but also the organizations you work for and the clients you serve. Luckily, burnout is something that you can avoid. In fact, most mental health professionals enjoy their profession and derive great purpose and meaning in what they do. Rather than focusing solely on prevention, it is best to focus on your own self-care as well. Effective self-care requires good self-awareness and self-monitoring. There are many proactive self-care strategies you can utilize: active and healthy body (exercising, eating, and sleeping well), active and healthy social life, rested and relaxed body and mind, spirituality, professional boundaries, personal mentor, and your own counselor. Although counseling can have its share of stressors, this does not mean that experiencing extreme emotional distress and possible burnout is a prerequisite to being a good counselor.

Chapter 7 addresses some of the more important components to developing and expanding your competency as a mental health counselor well after graduation and licensure. Regardless of your theoretical orientation, your effectiveness is linked to your level of competence. You have an ethical responsibility to monitor your effectiveness and build upon your skills when necessary. The following are some examples of core professional and personal areas to continually develop as a professional mental health counselor: practicing what you preach, considering counseling for yourself, receiving high-quality supervision, observing other counselors conduct sessions, continuing formal training after graduation (e.g., continuing education units), and embracing and accepting your anxieties and insecurities. Such training and development should be an integral component of your practice as long as you are in the profession.

Chapter 8 provides a review of some of the more necessary components to consider when starting a private practice. There is a good chance you have thought about starting your own private practice at some point in your graduate training. In most states, you will need to wait until you are independently licensed before this can become a realistic option. However, it is never too early to consider some of the components as you plan for your professional career as a mental health counselor. The content of this chapter is not meant as a "how to." Rather, this content is best viewed as information to consider as you make an informed decision toward having a private practice. This chapter considers the advantages and disadvantages to private practice, personal qualities associated with success, common mistakes, and the business aspect of private practice (e.g., financing, selecting a business entity, malpractice and business insurance, developing a business plan, financial planning, managed care organizations, marketing/advertising, and developing a niche for your practice). Starting a private practice can be quite challenging, but also extremely rewarding!

Acknowledgments

■ ■ ■

Thank you to Sophia DiDonna, my graduate research fellow, whose help in developing the state licensure table and converting my written documents into attractive electronic documents was invaluable. Thank you to Anthony Mastrocola and Anna Lindgren, my graduate research fellows, who significantly helped with revising and updating the state licensure table. Thank you to Zachary Aggott, MA, LMHC and Jacleen Charbonneau, MA, LMHC, my former students, who provided much assistance and key information for the discussion on teletherapy. Finally, thank you to Assumption University for my pre-tenure sabbatical. Without it, this book would have never happened.

I am most grateful for my wonderful wife, Yeonjoo Son. Her support and patience during the writing of this book and many other career accomplishments is greatly appreciated.

1

Is Being a Mental Health Counselor the Right Career Choice for You?

■ ■ ■

As you read this, you are probably already enrolled in a graduate program. So, you have already answered the question of whether being a mental health counselor is right for you! On the other hand, it is never too late for further introspection. Maybe you are having some ambiguous feelings as you learn the "ins and outs" of the mental health field during your internship. Or, maybe you are feeling confident in the path you are currently taking. Either way, it is my hope that this brief chapter will at least get you thinking about your key qualities and personal motivation for pursuing a career in counseling. Clinical mental health counseling is a demanding, but rewarding, profession that requires unique education and training. This is still an appropriate time in your professional development to contemplate the match between your personal goals, expectations, and values and what the field really has to offer.

WHY DO YOU WANT TO BE A MENTAL HEALTH COUNSELOR?

To help people. Those were probably the first words (or something similar) that came to your mind when you read the heading for this section. Why else would someone want to enter the profession of counseling? (Yes, a small percentage might have ulterior motives, but this is rare.) Some might want the secondary gain of personal benefit, but there is still the primary driving force to help others reduce their distress and improve their quality of life. A better question than "why" might be, "What is your motivation to be a counselor?" Perhaps you were inspired to help others like you were helped at an earlier stage of your life. Maybe the thought of being a healer by simply using your words is intriguing. Possibly, you have been told by many people that you are a good listener and provide helpful advice.

It is no secret that many (not all) counselors enter the field of counseling due to their own past personal mental health struggles and/or life challenges. There is nothing wrong with past experiences influencing one's current and future career aspirations. Being inspired to pursue a particular career path due to past experiences is not unique to the mental health field. However, what is unique is to be aware of how such past and current experiences can potentially influence the effectiveness of counseling. For example, your own personal experiences, values, and ways of coping with challenges most likely will differ from those of your clients. Additionally, some aspiring (and active) counselors hope that they can help themselves through their therapeutic relationship. Imposing your own values and trying to help yourself are damaging reasons to be a counselor. Counseling is not about you. It is about your clients. Thus, it is important to be aware of your own motivations to become a mental health counselor in order to ensure that you "are in it for the right reasons," for both your own benefit and that of your future clients.

Reflection Questions 1.1: Your Motivation to be a Mental Health Counselor

- Is your primary motivation to help others or yourself? If it is "yourself," what can you do to shift this motivation and self-monitor while working with clients?
- What are your motivations to become a counselor? Were there particular life events or people that inspired you to become a counselor?
- How can your personal motivations be a strength for your development as a counselor?
- What should you be aware of personally to ensure that your personal motivations do not interfere with effective counseling?

Of course, just like all human beings, counselors have personal needs. However, your personal needs should not impede your clients' growth. It is okay if you meet some of your needs through counseling in a secondary fashion. In other words, rather than pursuing personal growth as a primary gain, providing counseling in the best interests of your clients can result in significant personal growth. Counseling others can provide many personal and life perspectives and rewards that otherwise might not be experienced. This can be a catalyst for counselors to adaptively change over time. Overall, it is important to be aware of your own needs and know how to recognize if such needs are impacting the counseling relationship. If counseling is done appropriately, you can experience much personal growth without compromising your clients' well-being.

Reflection Questions 1.2: Balancing Your Personal Needs with Client Well-Being

- What are some of your personal needs? What are some ways in which such needs could interfere with counseling?
- How can you monitor your needs to avoid their interfering with the counseling relationship?
- What are alternative means to meet your unmet needs?
- What are some potential personal secondary rewards for counseling others?

Activity 1.1: Personal Qualities of Good Friends and Family vs. Mental Health Counselor

Before reading the next section, get into a small group of your peers and make a list of qualities that you like, or value, in your friends and family. Then, make a list of qualities that you think are necessary for good mental health counselors. Consider the following:

- What are the most important qualities that both groups of individuals have in common? What makes these qualities important?
- What are some qualities that are important for friends/family but not necessarily important for mental health counselors? Are these qualities simply not necessary for mental health counselors and/or could they be harmful?
- What are some qualities that are important for mental health counselors, but not necessary for family/friends? Why would these qualities not be necessary for friends/family?

WHAT ARE THE PERSONAL QUALITIES OF A MENTAL HEALTH COUNSELOR?

There are most definitely not just one or two (or more) types of mental health counselors. As you can probably tell from your peers in class and colleagues in internship, there are many different types of individuals that are counselors. This is a good thing. However many differences we may have in personal qualities and approaches to counseling, we have just as many, if not more, similarities. With that said, some personal qualities and approaches to counseling appear to enhance development of an adaptive and effective therapeutic relationship with clients (Duncan et al., 2010;

Kazantzis et al., 2017; Norcross, 2011). The following highlights some of the more common personal traits and approaches to counseling. Keep in mind that no counselor has all of the following traits. Thus, do not think of these personal qualities from an all-or-nothing perspective; rather, consider them on a continuum. Some qualities may be highly characteristic of you, at one extreme, and others may be very uncharacteristic of you at the other extreme. There may also be other qualities where you fall in the middle or are neutral.

Empathic with Compassion and Acceptance

Although seemingly obvious, it is vital that you are able to have empathy and compassion for your clients (Rogers, 1995). Empathy is the ability to put yourself in another person's shoes and understand their perspective. This allows you to understand and share the feelings and thoughts of your clients. You may not necessarily know exactly what their experiences are like, but you can at least understand their perspective. You can "feel" and cognitively understand their experience. Counselors are often taught that empathy is not the same as pity or compassion. This is true. Nevertheless, supplementing your empathy with compassion can go a long way in the healing process. By themselves, empathy and compassion generally do not produce long-term change. Yet, without empathy and compassion, counseling does not progress. Clients want to feel understood, or validated, for their experiences. They also do not want to be judged. Rather, they want to be accepted for who they are as human beings. The more comfortable clients feel with you, the more they will be willing to share their most distressing thoughts, emotions, and behaviors. And, the more they share such personal information, the more they can heal and grow. This sounds easy when initially learning about these terms and reading various case studies. However, even the most experienced counselors can be challenged at times. You will sometimes hear clients share some distressing/atypical thoughts and behaviors. Although empathy and compassion come naturally to most counselors, they are traits that evolve with experience and need to be continually monitored over time.

Genuine and Authentic

Counseling will make very little progress if you are not authentic to your clients and yourself (Rogers, 1995). In fact, if you cannot be authentic to yourself, it will be nearly impossible to be genuine to your clients. By looking at your own life and being honest with the changes you want to make, you model to your clients how to expose yourself and respond to life's challenges. In other words, effective counselors are congruent. If counselors are inauthentic, an adaptive working alliance will not be achieved. Counseling can be an intimate experience, which requires both parties to be true to themselves and each other. With that said, understandably, many clients will initially be hesitant to show their "true colors" until they feel more comfortable with you. The more you can be comfortable in your own skin, the more clients will show their own true colors. When both counselor and client are authentic with each other, the path for client growth (and counselor) is endless.

Dignity and Respect

All human beings deserve to be treated with dignity and respect. This includes how you treat yourself, the counselor. It is hard to treat others with dignity and respect if you cannot respect and appreciate yourself. Furthermore, dignity and respect is a reciprocal process. Where some people get stuck is waiting to receive respect before providing respect. This is a backwards way to approach life and counseling. Simply providing respect first often results in respect being reciprocated. Respecting your clients from the first time you interact with them conveys a sincere interest in their well-being and a desire to help. Eventually, most clients will reciprocate this respect through their conduct in counseling by actively engaging and being open to change by trying new ways of thinking and behaving.

Instill Hope

Effective counselors are able to instill hope for change in their clients (Coppock et al., 2010; O'Hara & O'Hara, 2012). In other words, they are good motivators. Clients often enter counseling under great distress. Many are at a loss as to what they can do to get better (that is why they are seeing you!), and some have lost any hope that anything will ever change. What is important to note here is that instilling hope requires being genuine in what is said and how it is conveyed. It would be unethical to lie to clients and say that "everything is going to be all right" or to promise you can "cure all their problems." Rather, you want to take factual information combined with your experience to communicate to your clients that you see potential for and are optimistic about improvement if effort is put into the process (on both sides). Simply validating their experience to seek help and appearing confident in your counseling skills is a strong step toward building hope and motivation to change.

Open and Tolerant

A competent counselor needs to be open and tolerant to those who have different backgrounds, world views, or ways of life (i.e., different cultures). These can include people of a different race, gender, age, sexual orientation, or social class. This does not mean you must agree with everything a client says or does. Rather, you will need to be both aware and comfortable with the fact that many of your clients will have different cultural backgrounds and life experiences than you. Some of these differences may be unique or shocking to you. Being open and tolerant with such differences starts with your own awareness of how your own culture affects you. This will allow you to respect the diversity of values espoused by clients from other cultures. Clients will notice this and soon come to feel more comfortable with someone who has a different background from them. Reciprocal modeling can occur where both counselor and client learn from each other's differences, which can ultimately result in a strong therapeutic alliance built upon trust and respect. (See the "Multicultural Awareness and Sensitivity" section below.)

Advocate and Empower

Occasionally your clients will come from a marginalized group or background that puts them at a significant social disadvantage for a variety of reasons. Although your primary responsibility is to provide effective counseling for your clients, this does not mean you cannot advocate for their well-being (Saliha & Blustein, 2018). Sometimes elements of your clients' distress cannot be resolved solely through counseling. In these cases, some of their distress may be due to external environmental factors that seemingly are out of your control. However, there may be appropriate opportunities where you can empower your clients to influence change, not just through motivation, but also through providing them appropriate resources outside of counseling. Social advocacy for your clients can also include getting involved in local community events or social justice issues at the local, state, or federal level. Only do what you feel comfortable with. What is important to recognize here is that there is potential to care and advocate for your clients beyond the counseling room.

Adaptive, Creative, and Flexible

To be an effective counselor, you will need to adapt to unexpected challenges that are not found in textbooks. This will require creativity and flexibility on your part (Owen & Hilsenroth, 2014). You will do your best as a graduate student to apply what you learned in class (and much reading and practice on your own) to your internship experiences. This is good. You need a solid foundation to start on. However, you will soon realize, if you have not already, that your clients' problems do not always fit the neat textbook case descriptions. This is where you will need to be creative in a way that still provides the best care possible for your clients, even if it is not a textbook approach to evidenced-based care. Furthermore, you will also have to learn how to work with colleagues from varying backgrounds (cultural and training) along with your agency and the mental health system. In this case, being adaptive will also include being flexible. You may notice a part of your agency or the mental health system that you do not like. However, you will soon learn that, in order to balance your own well-being and that of your clients, you will need to choose your battles. This by no means assumes complacency. Rather, it requires knowing what you are comfortable with accepting and what you believe is worth fighting for. Just like most professions, in counseling it is important to be ready and willing to adapt to the realities of the profession relative to your expectations and fantasies. Once the curtain to Oz is pulled back, what is seen cannot be unseen.

Acknowledge Weaknesses and Willing to Change

Effective counselors can acknowledge their weakness and mistakes and are willing to make necessary changes. This is not easy for most people. It requires a relatively strong ego and being secure with oneself. It takes much courage to admit you are not satisfied with yourself and to leave your comfort zone of baseline thinking and behaving. At first, evaluating your weaknesses, or personal flaws, may seem to be an intimidating task. However, with some practice, it can become more of a habit. In other words, the "sting" becomes less painful with each change. The point here is, how can you expect your clients to make changes in the way they think and behave if you do not do it yourself? This is where practicing what you preach becomes important. You do not have to be perfect at this; and it does not have to be easy. What is important is that you are open to improving yourself and make attempts at change. Ideally, you want to work toward being the person you want to become (i.e., "real self" to "ideal self"). It only makes sense that if you can model this to your clients, they will have a much better chance of working toward improving themselves as well. Also, your own personal experience with self-improvement can help you show empathy toward your clients when they struggle. If you reflect back on your own struggles, you will likely be less impatient and judgmental of your clients' hesitancies and mistakes.

Humor

Depending on your personality, you may either scoff at this quality or fully embrace it. Humor may be something you already use daily or something you are extra cautious with. In this context, it can simply mean not always taking everything too seriously and being able to "laugh at" (figuratively or literally) some of the daily nuisances that come with the profession. With a high-stress profession like clinical mental health counseling, your own well-being will benefit if you can sometimes go with the flow and brush off certain annoyances. Humor can help put life events in perspective. Humor can also help with your own mistakes and contradictions. Try to not take yourself too seriously and learn how to laugh at yourself. Additionally, if it does fit your personality, you can cautiously integrate some mild humor with counseling your clients (Gladding & Wallace, 2016). Of course, being humorous does not mean making fun of your clients, in session or out of session. Instead, a gentle joke about yourself or a client can lighten the mood. For example, pointing out with a little humor an unhelpful thought or behavior where no harm was done might bring attention to a bigger theme and potentially provide insight. In these cases, just make sure you have a solid therapeutic alliance and a good understanding of the client's personality.

Maintain Healthy Boundaries
Obviously, you want to make sure you maintain healthy boundaries with your therapeutic relationships. Ethically, your clients should always just remain your clients, nothing more. Here, maintaining healthy boundaries is more about the balance between being fully present for your clients in the moment while in session and yet not taking their problems home with you. This is a skill that is quite challenging for beginning counselors to acquire. Because counselors want to reduce their clients' distress and improve their well-being, almost inevitably they will have several clients that remain in their mind while having dinner with friends or watching a movie. It will take time and experience to learn the best way for you to provide high-quality care to your clients while keeping the rest of your day-to-day life separate. No counselor is perfect at this. A caveat here, especially for beginning counselors: some may feel guilty when they start to separate professional from personal life (e.g., "I just worked with a client with suicidal thoughts and now I'm enjoying dinner with my partner"). This also is normal and will subside over time. Look at it this way: just thinking about your client is not going to change any outcomes at this point. Furthermore, these thoughts are keeping you from being present with those who are closest to you; it is not fair to you or them. Allow yourself to focus your energy into other aspects of your personal life and be okay with it. (See Chapter 6 for a more extensive discussion on self-care and burnout.)

Present and Mindfully Oriented
A good personal and counseling skill is to be present-oriented, especially when focused on a particular task. In other words, being in the here and now helps you avoid getting stuck in the past or fixating on the future. A life with too many regrets or "what ifs" can result in much personal distress. If you spend too much time thinking about what could have been or what might happen, it takes away from your experience in the present, including

with those that are with you in the "now," like your clients. Eventually time passes and you have minimal experience or memories of the present. Try to practice being mindful by paying attention to your experiences in the present moment. Mindfulness also can be practiced through meditation. This is also a good skill to learn because it may eventually be one that you will want to teach your clients. Again, it is best to practice what you preach to be most effective with your clients.

Confident, Patient, and Grounded

To some degree, counselors are confident in their skills, patient while working with others, and grounded with regard to being well-balanced. As a beginning counselor, if you do not feel confident in your counseling skills, that is okay; you are still in the early stages of your professional development! If it helps, look at it more as being confident in knowing who you are and what you are capable of becoming. Others will notice this and respect it. Conversely, if you are confident in yourself, it is best to demonstrate patience and being grounded while working with others, especially those experiencing distress. Remember, in your role as a counselor, a key way to help others is by modeling through your own conduct. Being comfortable in your own skin and exuding confidence and patience across multiple contexts is quickly noticed by others.

Passionate and Enthusiastic

Having passion and enthusiasm to be effective at your profession is generally a must. (Of course, there can always be exceptions.) This appears to be especially true in the clinical mental health counseling field, as it can be associated with high levels of stress, including clients who are not always motivated to change and in whom such change can be hard to notice at times. Keep in mind, passion and enthusiasm do not have to mean that you run around your agency before each session yelling, "Yeah, let's go do some therapy!" Passion and enthusiasm can be experienced and expressed in many ways. In this case, it simply means having a strong desire to do things well while enjoying the process. Additionally, passion and enthusiasm add fuel to the fire of action. This is especially helpful when your energy is low and can be a strong protective factor against burnout.

Observe and Derive Satisfaction from the "Smaller Things"

Because clinical mental health counseling can be such a challenging profession, it is helpful to notice the "small things," or changes that our clients make. It is easy from session to session to get frustrated if clients are not making big, or at least observable, changes. The reality is that change often takes much time and effort. If you focus too much on your desired outcomes (e.g., what meeting all the treatment goals would look like), inevitably you will miss out on your clients' small steps toward self-improvement. The irony is that these small steps are where the true joy of counseling comes from, and not noticing them can impede client progress. For example, it is important that you notice minor improvement in your client's self-esteem, social skills, or simply how they present themselves (e.g., they are well groomed and smiling more). In other words, you want your clients to notice that you recognize such small changes. Validation, praise, and reinforcement can go a long way in increasing motivation and building upon change. If you can, try to derive meaning from such small changes in how you perceive your role in improving people's lives. It also helps to notice the small strides our profession makes in advocacy and gaining reputation and prestige among other related professions. Sometimes you can help improve the well-being of your clients through social advocacy. As you may guess, this type of change can take many years. There also currently appears to be a trend for greater recognition and appreciation for mental health services. Hopefully, this trend will continue as mental health stigma decreases and awareness of mental health issues increases.

Interpersonally Adept and Able to Connect

In short, having good interpersonal skills greatly enhances your ability to form therapeutic alliances and help clients change over time (Del Re et al., 2012). The sooner you can "connect" with your clients, the sooner you can use your therapeutic relationship to work on treatment goals. Ultimately, you want to build a collaborative relationship with your clients where you feel like you understand not only them but also their world. The reality is, no matter your theoretical orientation, your counseling skills will have limited effectiveness if you cannot use your interpersonal skills to connect with your clients. An especially important interpersonal skill for counseling is the ability to be self-aware (i.e., aware of how you come off to others). This requires considerable self-reflection, including being honest with yourself about your own weaknesses and biases. In the moment, self-awareness includes being able to adapt and "match" to your client in terms of verbal content, tone, modulated affect, physical mannerisms, and facial expressions. In other words, you cannot be 100% the same counselor for each client. It is vital that you are responsive to your clients' cognitive and emotional needs. You will learn over time how to modify both what you communicate and how you communicate (verbally and nonverbally) with each client. For example, some clients may prefer a slightly louder tone with more emotional expression, while others prefer a quieter one with more subtle expressiveness. Some clients may prefer humor in counseling, while you may never even consider using humor with other clients. Having the interpersonal skills to "read" your clients and to know both when and how to shift your approach with various clients will be greatly beneficial to the effectiveness of your counseling.

Activity 1.2: Your Mental Health Counselor Personal Qualities

Table 1.1 lists all the aforementioned personal qualities of a mental health counselor. It contains a scale (0–10; 0–not at all; 5–neutral or middle; 10–completely) to indicate how much you attribute each personal quality to yourself. There is also additional space to provide comments for each personal quality. What is most important is to give each quality some thought and to be honest with yourself. Upon completion of Table 1.1, get into a small group of peers and discuss the following reflection questions.

Table 1.1   Your Mental Health Counselor Personal Qualities

Personal Quality	Personal Rating (0–10) 0–not at all 5–middle or neutral 10–completely	Comments
1. Empathic with Compassion and Acceptance		
2. Genuine and Authentic		
3. Dignity and Respect		
4. Instill Hope		
5. Open and Tolerant		
6. Advocate and Empower		
7. Adaptive, Creative, and Flexible		
8. Acknowledge Weakness and Willing to Change		
9. Humor		
10. Maintain Healthy Boundaries		
11. Present and Mindfully Oriented		
12. Confident, Patient, and Grounded		
13. Passionate and Enthusiastic		
14. Observe and Derive Satisfaction from the "Smaller Things"		
15. Interpersonally Adept and Able to Connect		

- What personal qualities were the most surprising for you (i.e., surprised to rate yourself high, low, or neutral on a particular quality)?
- What personal qualities were the most confirming for you (i.e., ratings were what you expected)?
- What personal qualities are your greatest strengths? How will these strengths help you as a mental health counselor?
- What personal quality is your greatest weakness? Do you want to improve upon this quality? If so, how? If not, why?
- Regardless of your own ratings, what personal qualities do you think are a "must have" for mental health counselors?

SELF-AWARENESS OF AND COPING WITH PERSONAL ISSUES

Some of you may have had an initial interest in counseling and/or psychology because of curiosity about your own mental health and personal issues. This interest and curiosity may have motivated you to apply to graduate school to become a mental health counselor. Perhaps you have received help in the past and now want to help others. Perhaps you feel personally rewarded by helping others. Your motivations in pursuing a career in counseling could be an asset to your counseling skills. However, you should be aware, at the very least, of your own mental health status (Pieterse et al., 2013). In reality, all your personal issues will never be fully resolved. It is also possible to have some mental health struggles and still get by in life relatively well. Yet, if you are honest with yourself, you probably know when your mental health is impacting your daily life. If not, your mental health struggles could further extend into the quality of care you provide to clients. Not addressing your own mental health struggles will make it very difficult to adequately address your clients' mental health problems, especially if those are similar to yours. For example, if you present yourself as feeling hopeless, inevitably your clients will struggle to find hope in themselves to change. It is hard to ask something of your clients that you cannot do for yourself. If you think your mental health is impairing your daily functioning and/or your counseling skills, it is strongly suggested that you consider personal counseling (discussed more in Chapter 7). If it helps motivate you, consider that personal counseling is not just for yourself but also for the well-being of your clients. Ultimately, the main point here is not whether you are struggling with your mental health but how you are coping with it. Being a mental health counselor provides a unique opportunity for personal growth. Learning from your clients' transformative experiences and working on your own mental health can make you a better person and a better counselor. However, this will happen only if you directly address your own mental health and personal issues.

Reflection Questions 1.3: Self-Awareness and Insight of Personal Mental Health

- What personal mental health struggles and issues are you aware of? What are your thoughts about trying to alleviate some of this distress?
- What are some possible indicators that your mental health is impacting your daily functioning?
- What are some possible indicators that your mental health is impacting your client counseling skills?
- Do you have any personal mental health concerns that are impacting your ability to provide quality counseling? What are your options for addressing these concerns? Are you willing to consider mental health counseling for the benefit of both yourself and your clients?

MULTICULTURAL AWARENESS AND SENSITIVITY

A thorough discussion of multicultural competency in clinical mental health counseling is well beyond the scope of this book (see Ratts & Pedersen, 2014; Sue et al., 2019). Nevertheless, it is a topic worth highlighting as you pursue a career in counseling. Broadly defined, culture is the values, worldviews, customs, and behaviors shared by a particular group of people. Thus, culture is much more than race or ethnicity; it includes gender, age, sexual orientation, religion, socioeconomic status, and physical and mental functioning. A key component to being an effective counselor is being aware of the cultural diversity of your clients and how it influences your practice. You obviously are not expected to know all aspects of your clients' cultural backgrounds. However, try to practice humility while consistently pursing additional knowledge and trainings to build your competencies. Experiential learning also can be very powerful. When appropriate, you can ask clients to provide information about what they think are personally relevant aspects of their culture. Your own background also has shaped your worldview, which in turn influences how you perceive and respond to your clients, especially those with different backgrounds and worldviews. To ignore the role and influence of multicultural factors on counseling outcomes in your clients is poor practice. In fact, you have an ethical obligation to acquire an awareness and sensitivity to cultural differences to ensure that you are developing sound treatment plans and interventions that match the values of your clients. Your goal should be to help clients make changes in their life that are consistent with their worldview, not yours. If this is going to be a problem for you, counseling may not be your profession of choice.

A key part to being a multiculturally effective counselor is having an awareness and understanding of your own cultural background, including your own experiences, worldview, values, assumptions, biases, and prejudices (Pieterse et al., 2013; Sue et al., 2019). As difficult as it may be to acknowledge, we all have some biases and prejudices. If you think otherwise, you are not being honest with yourself or fair to your clients. The real concern here is failure to acknowledge these views and/or do anything about them. The quality of care provided to clients can be significantly compromised. In some cases, counseling can make clients worse if certain biases and prejudices are not addressed. It takes courage, vigilance, and perhaps some psychological pain to monitor and address your biases and prejudices; but it is worth it if you consider your own personal growth and the well-being of your clients.

Counselors should also be aware of how they are perceived by their clients, especially those from diverse cultures. Even if you as a counselor have no malicious intent, simply how you "look" or come off may affect how clients receive you and progress in counseling. Many of these factors are not your fault. You cannot control your race/ethnicity, gender, or age, for example. However, it is imperative to be aware of how your own cultural diversity can influence the counseling relationship. All counselors should be aware of how racism, sexism, ageism, heterosexism, ableism, socioeconomic factors, and other forms of discrimination and oppression can influence how clients perceive the world and their overall mental health. Depending on your background, you may have to consider if you have more privileges and entitlements than others (e.g., White, male, heterosexual, middle-class; Ivey et al., 2012). Having a different cultural background than your clients, including your privileges, does not mean it has to be problematic. Rather, being aware of these cultural differences allows you to be open (i.e., nondefensive), flexible, and ready to adapt accordingly. To not do so only perpetuates discrimination and fosters institutional racism (or any type of "ism").

Activity 1.3: Self-Awareness and Insight of Personal Cultural Privileges and Entitlements

Table 1.2 proposes some personal questions for reflection about your cultural background and associated privileges and entitlements, which may affect your counseling relationships. Do your best to be honest with yourself, even if you experience a little distress and defensiveness. Writing down and processing such thoughts typically provides greater personal clarity and reduces defensive thoughts, emotions, and behaviors. Upon completion of Table 1.2, get into a small group of peers to reflect upon your responses.

Table 1.2   Self-Awareness and Insight of Personal Cultural Privileges and Entitlements

How do you define your culture (e.g., gender, age, sexual orientation, religion, socioeconomic status, and physical and mental functioning)?	
What privileges and entitlements are associated with your cultural qualities?	
How could your privileges and entitlements affect the counseling relationship with your clients?	
What can you do to mediate the impact of your privileges and entitlements?	

In addition, consider the following questions.

- Were any of the questions difficult to answer (e.g., not sure how to define one's culture, struggle with awareness in identifying privileges or entitlements)?
- Did you experience any distressing thoughts or emotions when completing the questions? What could be some possible reasons for your reaction? What can be done about it?
- How would you describe your experience sharing your perceived cultural background and identified privileges and entitlements with others?
- What stereotypes or biases do you have that could potentially affect your counseling relationships? What can you do to work on these stereotypes and biases?
- What steps can you take to continue working on your multicultural competencies?

APPRECIATE THE IMPORTANCE OF SCIENCE: EVIDENCE-BASED PRACTICE

No matter your own personal approach to counseling, be sure to at least have the foundation of a theoretical approach supported by science. In other words, your case formulation, treatment goals, and especially interventions should be evidence-based. The field of clinical mental health counseling abounds with many amazing selfless human beings who put much effort into their practice and produce great long-term change in their clients. These individuals may vary in their approach to and style of utilizing their counseling skills, but what they do have in common is evidence-based practices.

Just doing what you think is right and going by "the gut," or even mystical forces, is not counseling. And, it is not good for your clients. Individuals who do not practice counseling with scientific underpinnings are not good for the field. Unfortunately, the field of counseling can also be a haven for such individuals because it is difficult to hold them accountable for what happens in the counseling room. Unlike other fields, incompetence in counseling (unless one is extremely bad at it!) may not be observed right away. Consequently, harm caused to clients by poor counseling can often be insidious and hard to notice. Consider two counselors: (1) poor in the counseling room, but great at completing paperwork; (2) great in the counseling room, but poor at completing paperwork. Ironically, it is the latter counselor that will get "caught" and put on notice before the former. This is because poor paperwork is often more noticeable than poor counseling. Over time, the former may get flushed out of the system, but not before harm has already been done to multiple clients. Also, unfortunately, some counselors are good at hiding their poor counseling skills for many years. The point here is that, unless you are audio/video supervised, nobody really knows what happens in the counseling room except for you and your clients. Thus, you have both a moral and an ethical obligation to provide the best possible care to your clients. This starts with using evidence-based interventions to build your competencies. No counselor is perfect. All counselors make mistakes. What is important is that you are true to yourself, knowing you do your best at helping your clients each day you practice.

Reflection Questions 1.4: Self-Awareness and Insight of Evidence-Based Practices

- What are your thoughts on using evidence-based practices with your clients?
- How can you balance your personal approach to counseling with using a theoretical approach based on science?
- What is some potential harm that can come from counselors who do not use evidence-based practices in the clinical mental health counseling field? What can be done to limit such individuals practicing in the field?

PUT THE EGO ASIDE: LEARN AS MUCH AS YOU CAN

From this day forward, promise yourself to put your ego aside and learn as much as you can from your professors, supervisors, colleagues, and any other experts you meet. This can be true of any profession, but it is especially salient for mental health counselors. You may already have many transferable skills, yet there is so much you do not know until you are exposed to it. Books on counseling skills are helpful and have their role. However, nothing can replace the guidance and expertise of professionals with many years of clinical experience. Experience matters a lot in this field. Also, if you are of a strong-minded nature, do your best to accept that, although you think you know a lot, there is much to be learned. Be humble. Having an unchecked ego can result in your being a poor counselor. The scary part is that poor counselors may think they are good counselors. These are the most dangerous type of counselors because they are oblivious to their incompetence and can cause the most damage to clients. So, check your ego at the door and take advantage of all the experts who want to use their time and energy to train you. Listen, watch, and learn. This will make you a better person and a competent mental health counselor. Counseling is truly a rewarding profession!

REFERENCES

Coppock, T. E., Owen, J. J., Zagarskas, E., & Schmidt, M. (2010). The relationship between therapist and client hope with therapy outcomes. *Psychotherapy Research, 20*, 619–626. http://dx.doi.org/10.1080/10503307.2010.497508

Del Re, A. C., Fluckiger, C., Horvath, A. O., Symonds, D., & Wampold, B. E. (2012). Therapist effects in the therapeutic alliance-outcome relationship: A restricted-maximum likelihood meta-analysis. *Clinical Psychology Review, 32*, 642–649. http://doi.org/10.1016/j.cpr.2012.07.002

Duncan, B., Miller, S. D., Wampold, B. E., & Hubble, M. A. (Eds.). (2010). *The heart and soul of change: Delivering what works in therapy* (2nd ed.). American Psychological Association.

Gladding, S. T., & Wallace, M. J. D. (2016). Promoting beneficial humor in counseling: A way of helping counselors help clients. *Journal of Creativity in Mental Health, 11*, 2–11. https://doi.org/10.1080/15401383.2015.1133361

Ivey, A., D'Andrea, M., & Ivey, M. (2012). *Theories of counseling and psychotherapy: A multicultural perspective* (7th ed.). Sage.

Kazantzis, N., Dattilio, F. M., & Dobson, K. S. (2017). *The therapeutic relationship in cognitive-behavioral therapy: A clinician's guide.* Guilford.

Norcross, J. C. (Ed.). (2011). *Psychotherapy relationships that work* (2nd ed.). Oxford University Press.

O'Hara, D. J., & O'Hara, E. F. (2012). Towards a grounded theory of therapist hope. *Counselling Psychology Review, 27*(4), 42–55.

Owen, J., & Hilsenroth, M. J. (2014). Treatment adherence: The importance of therapist flexibility in relation to therapy outcomes.
Journal of Counseling Psychology, 61, 280–288. https://doi.
org/10.1037/a0035753

Pieterse, A. L., Lee, M., Ritmeester, A., & Collins, N. M. (2013). Towards
a model of self-awareness development for counselling and psychotherapy training. *Counselling Psychology Quarterly, 26,* 190–
207. http://dx.doi.org/10.1080/09515070.2013.793451

Ratts, M. J., & Pedersen P. B. (2014). *Counseling for multiculturalism
and social justice: Integration, theory, and application* (4th ed.).
American Counseling Association.

Rogers, C. R. (1995). *On becoming a person: A therapist's view of psychotherapy.* Houghton Mifflin.

Saliha, K., & Blustein, D. L. (2018). Implementing social change: A
qualitative analysis of counseling psychologists' engagement in
advocacy. *The Counseling Psychologist, 46,* 154–189. https://doi.
org/10.1177/0011000018756882

Sue, D. W., Sue, D., Neville, H. A., & Smith, L. (2019). *Counseling the
culturally diverse: Theory and practice* (8th ed.). Wiley.

ADDITIONAL RESOURCES

Atkins, S. L., Fitzpatrick, M. R., Poolokasingham, G., Lebeau, M., &
Spanierman, L. B. (2017). Make it personal: A qualitative investigation of white counselors' multicultural awareness development. *The Counseling Psychologist, 45,* 669–696. https://doi.
org/10.1177/0011000017719458

Cook, A., & Miller, K. (2018). *Boundaries for your soul: How to turn
your overwhelming thoughts and feelings into your greatest allies.*
Thomas Nelson.

Duncan, B. L. (2010). *On becoming a better therapist.* American
Psychological Association.

Kottler, J. (2017). *On being a therapist* (5th ed.). Oxford University
Press.

Larsen, D. J., Stege, R., & Flesaker, K. (2013). "It's important for me not
to let go of hope": Psychologists in-session experiences of hope.
Reflective Practice, 14, 472–486. http://dx.doi.org/10.1080/14623
943.2013.806301

Larsen, D. J., Whelton, W. J., Rogers, T., McElheran, J., Herth, K.,
Tremblay, J., Green, J., Dushinski, K., Schalk, K., Chamodraka, M.,
& Domene, J. (2020). Multidimensional hope in counseling and
psychotherapy scale. *Journal of Psychotherapy Integration, 30,*
407–422. http://dx.doi.org/10.1037/int0000198

Singh, A. A., Appling, B., & Trepal, H. (2020). Using multicultural and social justice counseling competencies to decolonize counseling practice: The important roles of theory, power, and action. *Journal of Counseling and Development, 98*, 261–271. https://doi.org/10.1002/jcad.12321

Wampold, B. E., & Imel, Z. E. (2015). *The great psychotherapy debate: Models, methods, and findings* (2nd ed.). Lawrence Erlbaum Associates.

2

Professional Identity Development and Ethics

■ ■ ■

Although this chapter is treated as two separate sections, professional identity development and professional ethics are naturally integrated topics. The review of these topics is not meant to be exhaustive. There are separate texts with multiple extensive chapters that solely cover professional identity development and professional ethics (see Corey et al., 2019; Granello & Young, 2019). The focus of this chapter is to provide a relatively brief overview of these two topics while highlighting the most relevant points within the scope of preparing to be a professional mental health counselor. In other words, the review here of professional identity development and professional ethics provides a guiding foundation for the remaining chapters in this text (e.g., self-care and burnout, obtaining a job, developing therapy skills). Not being cognizant of your developing professional identity and a lack of awareness of key ethical foundations makes the remaining chapters in this book moot.

PROFESSIONAL IDENTITY DEVELOPMENT

Defining and establishing a professional identity is a continuous process for all professions. A strong professional identity is important for a profession to succeed, advance, and establish prestige over time. Ideally, mental health counselors with a strong professional identity should be able to accurately describe their graduate program, accreditation, and associated approach to practice; identify their qualifications, areas of expertise, and licensing credentials; identify and explain key similarities and differences between their profession and other similar professions; and have a sense of belonging among other mental health counselors. Furthermore, professional identity development plays a central role in establishing and maintaining sound ethical practice (see Corey et al., 2019; Granello & Young, 2019).

Professional identity is an especially nebulous concept for mental health counselors due to varying backgrounds in education; different accreditation, professional memberships, and state licensing bodies; varying roles/duties; much overlap with similar professions; and relatively short established history. These professional development and practice factors greatly contribute to the lack of collective identity among mental health counselors. Perhaps there will always be at least some variation in professional identity among mental health counselors (see American Counseling Association [ACA], Council for Accreditation of Counseling and Related Education Programs [CACREP], American Mental Health Counselors Association [AMHCA], Masters in Psychology and Counseling Accreditation Council [MPCAC]). Having multiple professional organizations (e.g., ACA and AMHCA) and multiple accrediting bodies (e.g., CACREP and MPCAC) may actually have more benefits than drawbacks for the profession of mental health counselors. Such diversity in training can have the added value of expanding the quality of mental health care for the public good, as long as evidence-based practices are utilized.

The following discussion of professional identity will not be a history of a specific field or type of program. Such information does have relevance, but it is best left up to each specific program and other texts that primarily focus on history. Developing a collective identity based on history and philosophies is not advocated for either. Rather, what may be the most important is how you integrate your personal attributes/identity and professional training within the context of professional practice and community. With that said, even those from different training, accreditation, and professional membership backgrounds have many more commonalities than differences.

Education and Accreditation

The required education level for mental health counselors is a master's degree. Clinical social work and psychiatric nursing also both require a master's degree. Psychologists require a doctoral degree (e.g., Ph.D. or Psy.D.), and psychiatrists require a medical degree (M.D.). A master's degree that leads to licensure as a mental health counselor can come from a variety of graduate programs: mental health counseling, clinical mental health counseling, clinical community mental health, counseling psychology, clinical psychology, clinical-counseling psychology, applied psychology, school counseling, and counselor education. Although there will be some curriculum differences related to program name/degree (e.g., clinical-counseling psychology vs. counselor education) and accreditation (e.g., CACREP or MPCAC), the required core content for state requirements for licensure will have more similarities. (See Chapter 3 for a more detailed discussion about education and licensure requirements.)

The two most common professional associations associated with mental health counselors are the ACA and AMHCA. Until recently (April, 2019), AMHCA used to be a division of ACA, but they are now separate associations. Of course, there are many different types of counselors across the nation. However, AMHCA was charged with supporting the needs of mental health counselors. On the other hand, ACA focuses on all counselors across multiple specialties (e.g., rehabilitation counselors, school counselors, employment counseling). Currently, as a stand-alone association, AMHCA is the only one that is "uniquely dedicated to the academic, internship, supervision, and licensure of mental health counselors. AMHCA supports students, faculty, supervisors, supervised pre-licensed and licensed clinical mental health counseling professionals" (AMHCA, 2019). AMHCA and ACA will continue to work together on mental health issues and topics of mutual interest. Of course, counselors solely affiliated with ACA can often still get their professional needs met. There may be other counselors who are affiliated with both ACA and AMHCA. Understandably, as with having different training and accreditation backgrounds, it can be hard to develop a collective identity with different professional associations representing the "same" group of mental health counselors. Some may argue that it is best for training programs to "choose" one membership over another (similar to accreditation). Others may argue that it is best for students to choose one or both based upon their individual professional needs and goals. Regardless of membership, there are often more similarities than differences due to similar professional interests.

Overall, the closest approach toward collective identity seems to come from state licensure, at least with respect to required curriculum, professional recognition, and reimbursement from managed care. Thus, regardless of whether you graduate from a clinical-counseling psychology or counselor education program, or your program is CACREP accredited or MPCAC accredited, you are on the same "professional team." Your professional identity should at least be similar with regard to goals for the profession, including advocacy and legislation (e.g., vs. licensed social workers or licensed psychologists). In the end, it is more productive for same-licensed individuals to work together through their similarities and mutual interests rather than focus on their differences.

Scope and Approach to Practice

The specific activities that counselors can engage in is based upon "scope of practice," a common term used by licensure boards to describe the rights and limitations of any practicing profession. This includes the clients served by the practicing profession, including necessary procedure and processes. Licensure boards determine the scope of practice for mental health counselors, which then becomes state law. Because of this, scope of practice for mental health counselors varies by state. With that said, there is much similarity in scope of practice throughout the states. In most states, in addition to mental health counseling, mental health counselors are able to engage in assessment (intake and many other formal assessments), diagnostic evaluation, and case management. The populations served with these activities include individuals, families, couples, and groups. Most mental health counselors engage in other activities such as teaching and advocacy. Be sure to research your state law to know the licensure requirements, professional title of your license to practice, and scope of practice, including limitations. (See Chapter 3 for a more extensive discussion about licensure.) Also, keep in mind that mental health counselors work with many other mental health professionals in related fields (e.g., social workers, psychologists, psychiatrists) and engage in many of the same activities as other professionals do. However, the service provided by itself is not fully indicative of one's professional identity. Rather, the training philosophy, professional membership, and theoretical orientation are more representative of one's professional identity.

It can be a challenge to identify what distinguishes clinical mental health professionals from other mental health professions. In the late 1970s, professional mental health counseling was defined as "an interdisciplinary multifaceted, holistic process of (1) the promotion of healthy life-styles, (2) identification of individual stressors and personal levels of functioning, and (3) preservation or restoration of mental health" (Seiler & Messina, 1979, p. 6). In other words, many mental health counselors espouse the wellness and strength-based model over the medical model (Mellin et al., 2011; Myers et al., 2000), which is more commonly associated with psychologists and psychiatrists. While the wellness and strength-based model focuses on enhancing strengths to maximize potential, the medical model views emotional distress as an illness that requires "curing" from a diagnostic perspective. Additionally, the wellness and strength-based model views mental health distress as a part of normal development, taking into account life stages. There is also a stronger emphasis on prevention and early intervention rather than curing, which can include empowerment. On the other hand, the medical model primarily first focuses on identifying problems from a pathology perspective. These different perspectives can clearly result in how clients' emotional distress and problems are conceptualized and treated, including goals and interventions. The wellness and strength-based model can be a helpful component to mental health counselors' professional identity. However, be aware that other mental health professionals would also state they subscribe to this approach (i.e., not all psychologists or psychiatrists strictly follow the medical model). Furthermore, even mental health counselors who strongly subscribe to the wellness and strength-based model will still need to be well versed in the medical model, as this is an inherent part of the mental health care system, including working with managed care organizations.

Specialization, Population Served, and Setting

It is okay if you do not follow a specific identity model. Mental health counselors all have personal attributes, unique backgrounds, and great variety in their education and training. Furthermore, specialization (e.g., addiction, trauma, eating disorders), population served (e.g., adolescents, veterans, geriatric), and setting (e.g., outpatient, school, hospital) are significant factors in counselor identity development (Myers et al., 2002). Professional identity is unique to each individual. With that said, in addition to your professional organization affiliations (e.g., ACA or AMHCA), knowing your scope of practice and employing the wellness and strength-based model can be a good start to the foundation of your professional identity. This can also help mental health counselors find at least some common ground across a very diverse group of professionals. A key aspect of your professional identity is to be continuously mindful of how your professional (decisions, roles, ethics) and personal (perceptions, values, morals) selves evolve over time (Auxier et al., 2003). Ultimately, your professional identity will greatly influence your thoughts, emotions, and behaviors, including how you perceive and treat your clients.

Intrapersonal and Interpersonal Dimensions

As a beginning mental health counselor, your professional identity development includes intrapersonal and interpersonal dimensions (Gibson et al., 2010). The intrapersonal dimension includes integrating your personal identity with the identity of the profession (i.e., personal and professional selves). This includes transitioning from external authority figures and experts (e.g., professors) to authorities in the profession (e.g., clinical supervisors). Over time, this includes embracing professional values, ethics, attitudes, roles, skills, and ways of thinking and solving problems (Auxier et al., 2003). Of course, your perception of the identity of the profession will be greatly influenced by those you work closest with (e.g., colleagues, clinical supervisor, agency) and obtaining real counseling experience with clients. The interpersonal dimension includes receiving and processing feedback from other more experienced professionals as attempts are made to enter and assimilate into the professional culture of clinical mental health counseling (Dollarhide & Miller, 2006; O'Byrne & Rosenberg, 1998). Here, new information is compared with previous understandings, evaluated,

and either intergraded or rejected. These two processes co-occur in a reciprocal fashion. In other words, development in one dimension will influence
development in the other dimension. You will notice that your professional
identity development will include a continuous cycle of learning, practice,
and feedback while experiencing both autonomy and dependence. This process is often associated with initial self-doubt and anxiety. Ultimately, a key
indicator that your professional identity is "mature" is when you notice
increasing self-efficacy and that your locus of evaluation and validation is
primarily internal.

Activity 2.1: Personal Professional Identity

Figure 2.1 provides a visual diagram of the aforementioned components of
professional identity. This review was by no means exhaustive; its focus was
to highlight some of the more salient components of professional identity
to stimulate personal reflection. Review Figure 2.1 and consider your own
definition of professional identity development, including any additional
components you think should be included. You can also rank or use a scale
(0–10) to determine your personal value (or weight) for each of the components, including additional components you may have added. Thereafter, get
into a small group of peers and discuss the following reflection questions.

- Of the listed professional identity components, which ones resonate
  with you the most (perhaps based on your ranking or scale)? Which
  personal identity elements resonate with you the least?
- What other components not listed are personally important to your
  professional identity (consider theoretical orientation [an emphasis
  on your master's degree training], use of empirically supported
  interventions, significant individuals or life events, or your personal
  background/culture)?
- What would be your own personal definitions of professional identity
  development?
- What distinguishes your identity from other professions (i.e., between-
  group differences)?
- What distinguishes your identity from those of other people in your
  own profession of clinical mental health counseling (i.e., within-group
  differences)?

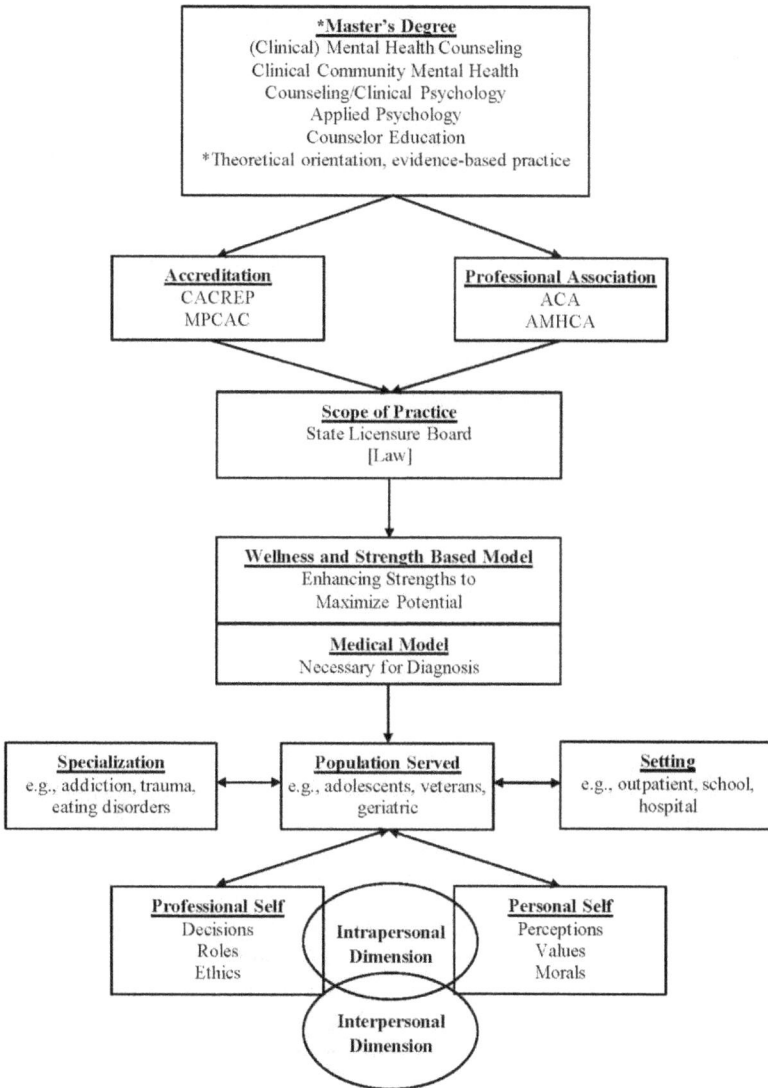

Figure 2.1 Professional Identity Development Components

PROFESSIONAL ETHICS

In many ways, within the context of this chapter, professional ethics could be treated as a subheading to professional identity development. As discussed earlier, a key contributing factor to professional identity is affiliation with professional organizations like ACA or AMHCA, both of which have their own separate codes of ethics. Following your professional membership's code of ethics can very much shape your professional identity, as it is something you must first become familiar with during your graduate training and then throughout your professional career. Nevertheless, a discussion of ethics for mental health counselors requires its own unique focus.

You have most likely already taken (or will soon take) a graduate course in ethics, as this is required by all state licensing boards. Thus, the focus of this section is on the broad principles of ethics most relevant to mental health counselors. It will not be a detailed overview of all the codes of ethics, which is well beyond the scope of this chapter and text (See Corey et al., 2019). The basics of and relationship between values, morals, ethics, and laws will be reviewed. Thereafter, the importance of professional organizations having codes of ethics, like ACA and AMHCA, will be discussed. Ethical decision-making and legal issues relevant to counseling will be highlighted. Finally, concluding comments will be made about how to ensure that you maintain ethical practice.

Defining: Values, Morals, Ethics, and Laws

It is important to differentiate the terms values, morals, ethics, and laws. Broadly speaking, values come from within ourselves and are beliefs and attitudes that we have about everyday life which influence our choices (i.e., thoughts) and behaviors. Some values are weighted more than other values based upon our own personal experiences and can change over time. Values give our lives meaning. Morals are our personal belief system, which focuses on what we perceive to be right and wrong conduct. Morals are typically influenced by our values and cultural and/or religious/spiritual standards (i.e., society), which in turn influence the lens through which we evaluate the actions/conduct of ourselves and others. Morals are more deep-seated than values within individuals but can vary between individuals and across cultures. While morals are personal codes, ethics are codes followed by a group by blending values and morals in order to constitute rules for right conduct. Codes of ethics are developed by professional organizations to inform their members on moral behaviors and moral decision-making. Ethics can evolve over time to reflect changes in society and the profession. It is expected that the members of an organization follow its code of conduct. If not, there can be consequences ranging from a reprimand to termination of membership. Laws are related to rules determined through society (e.g., legislation in the U.S.) that address proper conduct on how individuals should live together. While codes of ethics are created by members of a professional organization, laws are created by elected officials. Ethics are enforced and interpreted by ethics committees and licensing/certification boards. Laws are enforced by police and interpreted by judges. Breaking a law is always a criminal offense. Sometimes unethical behaviors can also be illegal. From a practicing mental health counselor perspective, look at laws as a minimum level of practice and ethics as an ideal level of practice. Ultimately, it appears that your moral development is a significant predictor of your professional ethical identity development (Lloyd-Hazlett & Foster, 2016)

The Necessity for Having an Established Code of Ethics

A formal code of ethics helps a profession legitimize its professional status. All mental health professions (e.g., counseling, social work, psychology, psychiatry) have well-established codes of ethics to provide their members guidelines on how to behave (or not behave) and make moral decisions. At first thought, you might be curious as to why codes of ethics are even necessary for a profession that is dedicated to serving those experiencing distress. Who would want to hurt those they are trying to help? Being a mental health counselor appears to be an inherently ethical profession. In most cases this is quite true. However, a profession that works closely with vulnerable populations needs to develop and uphold a code of ethics in order to set minimum professional standards of practice, also known as mandatory ethics. Having a formal code of ethics educates counselors and clients about what constitutes ethical practice, which ensures accountability that protects and promotes the welfare of clients. Most counselors would not deliberately harm their clients. However, unfortunately, like all professions, a few individuals could engage in conduct that harms clients. Furthermore, most ethical dilemmas are not directly related to deliberately harming clients. Rather, a code of ethics should act as a guide to help well-intentioned counselors make sound moral decisions. Doing what is in the best interest of clients is known as aspirational ethics. Note that ethics rarely provides an explicit answer. Instead, there are often multiple answers, and counselors must choose the one they believe is most appropriate. Relatedly, a code of ethics also protects counselors. By demonstrating that well-thought-out decisions were made by following a profession's code of ethics, counselors are generally protected from public and legal scrutiny (i.e., licensing board complaint or malpractice suit). This process also allows for the profession to self-regulate autonomously rather than be overseen by the government.

Although there can be differences between professional organizations' codes of ethics, there are often more similarities. With that said, due to possible multiple professional memberships, there can sometimes be multiple codes of ethics within a profession, including mental health counselors. Furthermore, state regulatory boards can vary by what codes of ethics they follow and/or may have their own independent code of ethics. There can also be areas of specialization within a profession that may require additional guidelines. The focus of the remainder of this chapter is on the two codes that apply to most mental health counselors across all 50 states: the ACA Code of Ethics (ACA, 2014) and the AMHCA Code of Ethics (AMHCA, 2020).

The current ACA Code of Ethics was most recently revised in 2014, and the current AMHCA Code of Ethics was most recently revised in 2020. Recall from the discussion earlier in this chapter that AMHCA used to be a division of ACA until April 2019. This means AMHCA and ACA are two separate associations. ACA focuses on all counselors, regardless of specialty. AMHCA focuses solely on mental health counselors. Thus, it is not unreasonable to assume that you are (or will be) a member of at least one of these professional associations, or possibly both.

Both associations have revised their codes of ethics multiple times. This is to be expected. Codes of ethics are living documents that are periodically reviewed and modified over time. Typically, the fundamental components of each ethical principle do not change, but new issues and questions arise related to the practice of counseling in response to society. Examples include a growing awareness of multicultural factors, societal/social justice changes, and even technology. For example, when the use of computers became common practice for counselors, there were ethical concerns about client information stored on computers. Now there are concerns about internet counseling (i.e., teletherapy) and managing relationships with clients or supervisees on social media.

The stated purposes of the ACA Code of Ethics and the AMHCA Code of Ethics are very similar. Both codes emphasize the importance of their use to define ethical behaviors and as a guide to assist members to make sound ethical decisions. Both codes explicitly state that the codes are not only for current and prospective members, but also for the public at large, including those served/clients. Lastly, the codes make note of supporting the mission of their associations.

The ACA Code of Ethics contains nine main sections in the following areas: the counseling relationship; confidentiality and privacy; professional responsibility; relationships with other professionals; evaluation, assessment, and interpretation; supervision, training, and teaching; research and publication; distance counseling, technology, and social media; and resolving ethical issues. The AMHCA Code of Ethics contains six main sections with multiple subsections that address the following areas: commitment to clients (counselor–client relationship; counseling process; counselor responsibility and integrity; assessment and diagnosis; record keeping, fee arrangements, and bartering; other roles); commitment to other professionals (relationships with colleagues, clinical consultation); commitment to students, supervisees, and employee relationships (relationships with students, interns, and employees; commitment for clinical supervision); commitment to the profession (teaching, research and publications, service on public or private boards and other organizations); commitment to the public (public statements, marketing); resolution of ethical problems. The content of both codes of ethics is very similar. The only marked difference between both codes is that AMHCA devotes a significantly greater amount of detail to working with clients in a clinical context. This makes sense, considering AMHCA's sole commitment to representing mental health counselors while ACA represents counselors across multiple disciplines.

Overall, based upon ACA's and AMHCA's preambles, purposes, and codes of ethics there are a few broad similar themes as well: primary consideration for the welfare of clients; avoiding harm and exploitation; safeguarding confidentiality (practice, teaching, or research); respecting the dignity and rights of clients, including avoiding discrimination; only practicing within the scope of one's competence; overall adherence to ethics; and representing the association and profession with integrity while striving for aspirational practice.

A common and understandable thought is, "as a mental health counselor, which code do I fall under?" An initial response is, "it depends." In other words, it truly depends on your professional affiliation. If you are a member of only ACA or AMHCA, then you should follow that affiliation's code of ethics. On the other hand, if you are a member of both ACA and of AMHCA, you technically fall under both codes. However, in this case, as a mental health counselor you may find AMHCA's code more representative of your specialty. This is because not only does AMHCA's code incorporate all the core values and principles of ACA's code, it provides more direct guidance to working with clients in a clinical context. With all of that said, you will also have to take state law into consideration. Each state can make an independent choice to adhere to ACA, AMHCA, and/ or state-specific codes. Because AMHCA has a primary focus on mental health counselors, many states choose the AMHCA code. However, many states also use ACA's code as the primary code for all counselors, especially because AMHCA used to be a division of ACA until April 2019. There are other states that adhere to both codes. There are a few states that do not explicitly adhere to ACA or AMHCA codes due to following state-specific codes. Finally, there are also some states that adhere to one or both codes while also including additional state-specific codes. Additionally, if you are seeking credentialing, such as National Certified Counselor (NCC), you will also have to adhere to the National Board for Certified Counselors (NBCC) code. Finally, you may also choose to obtain additional certifications (e.g., Certified Substance Abuse Counselor), which also may have its own code of ethics. In the end, it is your responsibility to be aware of the codes for your professional memberships and certifications, and/or state-specific codes. From a pragmatic standpoint, although it is important to morally follow all codes of ethics associated with your memberships and certifications, from a legal liability standpoint you must ensure that you follow the codes of the states you practice in.

Reflection Questions 2.1: Getting to Know Your Code of Ethics

- What are some ways mental health counselors could unintentionally harm their clients? What can you do in your own practice to minimize the chances of such unintentional harm?
- Knowing that codes of ethics are living documents, what are some current or new issues that should be addressed in the practice of counseling?
- Do you have a membership with ACA and/or AMHCA? Are you familiar with their codes of ethics? Do you know what state you want to practice in and what code of ethics it follows? Do you (or will you) belong to another credentialing body or have (or will have) any additional certifications that have their own code of ethics? What can you do to know which codes of ethics to follow and begin to apply them to your practice?

Ethical Decision-Making

The focus of this discussion is not on solving specific ethical dilemmas, as this is reserved for ethics courses. However, it is important to be aware that many ethical decision-making models exist, but no single model has been shown to be universally effective across all dilemmas. The goal here is to highlight some of the most common components in many of these ethical decision-making models. This information should provide perspective on what needs to be considered and the types of thought processes when making ethical decisions. As stated earlier, codes of ethics do not tell you what decision to make for a specific ethical dilemma. They are only the beginning part of the ethical decision-making process. In other words, codes of ethics are necessary but not sufficient for making ethical decisions.

Rather, they are guides to aid in your decision-making. Ethical dilemmas are very complex and unique to each situation. Your own ethical knowledge and awareness, problem-solving skills, and decision-making model will be your driving force in recognizing, contemplating, and responding to ethical dilemmas.

Both the ACA and AMHCA codes of ethics state that counselors should utilize an ethical decision-making process when an ethical dilemma is encountered. It is important to understand the primary underlying moral principles for many of these ethical decision-making models (see Beauchamp & Childress, 2012; Kitchener, 1984; Meara et al., 1996). In fact, the Preamble to the ACA Code of Ethics includes six moral principles: (1) autonomy (clients have the ability to choose; self-determination), (2) nonmaleficence (do not harm clients), (3) beneficence (do good and help clients), (4) justice (treat clients fairly and equitably), (5) fidelity (be loyal and honor commitments to clients; trustworthy); (6) veracity (truthfulness and honesty with clients). All of these principles should be valued equally and concurrently considered when faced with making an ethical decision. However, each individual incident may result in competing principles, where one is weighed more than another. For example, a suicidal client may need to be involuntarily hospitalized (reduced autonomy) in order to avoid harm and do good (nonmaleficence and beneficence).

Although you may come to adhere to a particular ethical decision-making model(s) as you gain more counseling experience, here it is beneficial to understand some of most effective components of these models. Corey et al. (2019) provide a great a stepwise procedure that can be used for most (if not, all) ethical dilemmas. The following summarizes the key components of each step:

1. *Dilemma identification.* Gather as much information as possible to be sure that there truly is a problem or dilemma. Is this a situation that is truly ethical in nature? It could also be a moral, legal, clinical, or professional issue (or a combination). This is where you should begin documenting your thought processes, decisions, and any actions taken.
2. *Potential issues identification.* Take into consideration the welfare of all individuals that may be affected by the situation, including their rights and responsibilities. Consider the context of the situation, including such factors as culture, race/ethnicity, religious/spiritual background, age, socioeconomic status, and relationships (including power and privilege).

3. *Review the appropriate ethics codes.* This will give you initial guidance on how to move forward. Do your best to be self-aware of how well your own values and morals match with the relevant ethics codes (i.e., consider any potential conflict). Do any of the ethics codes provide guidance in developing a solution to the dilemma? It is important to document this process to highlight your concerted effort to adhere to relevant ethics codes.

4. *Review the appropriate laws and regulations.* Also consider the relevant rules and regulations of your agency. Consider how any laws and regulations have relevance to the ethical dilemma. Again, document this process.

5. *Consult with other professionals.* Talking to other professionals that are more experienced and come from different perspectives (perhaps neutral) can provide more objectivity and insight. It is also prudent to document what suggestions you received from your consultations.

6. *Formulate possible action plans.* This includes continuing your discussions with other professionals for possible options on how to respond to the ethical dilemma. Ideally, try to identify multiple options while considering ethical and possible legal implications. If relevant and appropriate, consider including the client(s) in this process. Be sure to document these discussions, especially any with a client.

7. *Consider the consequences for each action plan.* In other words, what are the implications if you were to follow through with each action plan? You should consider how your client(s), others involved, and yourself will be impacted by any action taken. This includes potential risks and benefits (physical and psychological) to all individuals involved. Also, consider practicality with regard to time, effort, and resources. If reasonable, the consequences for each action plan should be discussed with your client(s).

8. *Choose the best action plan.* After implementation of your action plan, evaluate the outcomes on all individuals involved. Thereafter, determine if additional action must be taken. Finally, document the rationale for your actions and your evaluation process (and any additional actions).

With most ethical dilemmas, it is rare that only one course of action is required. Sometimes these steps are not linear and have to be repeated after evaluating your initial course of action. As noted in the steps, be sure to maintain accurate and clear documentation throughout the decision-making process. In the end, self-reflection and evaluating outcomes with those you consulted with can build upon your ethical decision-making skills.

Reflection Questions 2.2: Reflecting on Making Ethical Decisions

- Considering ACA's six moral principles (i.e., autonomy, nonmaleficence, beneficence, justice, fidelity, and veracity), what are some other possible examples of incidents where these principles may compete? How do you know when to weigh one principle more than another?
- What are your thoughts on using an ethical decision-making model? What components of an ethical decision model may be the most challenging for you to complete?
- What are your initial thoughts and feelings when considering that most ethical dilemmas rarely have only one course of action? Is it possible to have multiple courses of action where all have a desired outcome?

Legal and Ethical Issues in Counseling

Although codes of ethics are designed for mental health counselors to "self-govern," the law must still be followed. Both the ACA and AMHCA codes of ethics explicitly state that counselors must follow relevant federal and state laws. Developed through society, laws are a minimum standard accepted by society. There are times when counselors engage in unethical behavior that is also illegal. There are other times when counselors may be asked to assist in the legal process (e.g., subpoena to testify in court). In almost all circumstances (e.g., court case), the law typically overrules ethics. Not surprisingly, there can be vast discrepancies across state laws. The obvious conclusion to make here is that it is your responsibility to know not only relevant codes of ethics, but also relevant state and federal laws.

With some ethical dilemmas, there is little to no conflict between ethics and the law. In these cases, either the ethics and law are compatible or you are comfortable with the law that overrules ethics. Of course, there may be times when there appears to be conflict between your code of ethics and the law. Ideally, being proactive to anticipate possible problems can help minimize these conflicts. However, this is not always possible or practical. You now have a dilemma between ethics and law about how to handle an ethical dilemma. This is when your values and morals are more explicitly taken into consideration. The most common scenario is when following your code of ethics could potentially result in breaking the law. Your options often include following the law in a way that minimizes harm to ethics or adhering to ethics in a way that minimizes breaking the law. In either case, it is best to seek legal advice and consult with your state licensing board. Do not handle these ethical dilemmas without consulting a legal expert. This will not only aid you in your decision but also protect you and your client(s).

If you behave unethically, you could be reported to the state licensing board by one of your clients (or clients' relatives) and/or colleagues. The state licensing board will then conduct an investigation to determine if the allegations are true. If it is determined you have engaged in unethical behavior the board will move forward with a disciplinary hearing. Possible repercussions vary by state and severity of unethical behavior: (1) verbal/written reprimand/warning, (2) put on probation with the requirement to take courses/trainings, (3) license suspended with the requirement to take courses/trainings to remove suspension, (4) termination of your license. Depending on the severity of the unethical behavior, there may be an option to reapply for licensure in the future, which may also require additional courses/trainings. In addition to state licensing boards, ACA and AMHCA (and other professional organizations) have ethics committees. The primary roles of these ethics committees are to revise and update their organization's code of ethics, educate its members about their code of ethics, and protect the public from unethical behavior. Clients and/or colleagues can also file a formal complaint to the organization(s) you belong to. The ethics committees will then process the formal complaint against you to determine if you engaged in an unethical behavior. The committees can decide to either dismiss the complaint or move forward with sanctions if it is determined you behaved unethically. Responses can range from a warning/reprimand to probation/suspension with required remedial action (e.g., courses/trainings in ethics) to being expelled. It is important to note that disciplinary action by state licensing boards and organization ethics committees are two separate entities and processes. In other words, one could lose their organization membership, but will receive consequences from the state licensing board only if an independent investigation is conducted as a result of a separate complaint.

If you engage in illegal behavior, you could be prosecuted in a criminal court (e.g., insurance fraud or physical assault), which can include being punished with a monetary fine and/or incarceration in jail or prison. There can also be civil lawsuits (e.g., breaking confidentiality, inappropriate interventions; typically less severe and not necessarily illegal; lower threshold for confidence in guilt), which is a way to compensate (usually monetarily) the client victim for being wronged. Although you cannot control everything, you can certainly minimize the chances of behaving unethically or breaking the law. In addition to knowing your professional codes of ethics and state statutes, you should always treat clients with dignity and respect while keeping their welfare a primary concern.

Being a mental health counselor does carry a certain level of risk. Most counselors are good people who would never deliberately behave unethically or break the law. However, minor mistakes can happen (the bigger types of mistakes are more likely deliberate), and sometimes you can be accused of something you truly did not do. No counselor is exempt from the possibility of being criminally charged or a lawsuit. Therefore, you should always carry professional liability insurance to protect yourself from your actions or accusations of actions. Always be prepared for the unexpected. Such coverage is a relatively small price for protecting against a potential big career and/or financial cost. If you are a student counselor and a member of ACA or AMHCA, you can receive free liability insurance. This is most helpful while doing your practicum and internship. In addition, keep in mind that during your training (including until you are licensed) you also fall under your supervisor's license. Thus, you also have the ethical (and moral) responsibility to conduct yourself in a professional manner, as you could negatively affect not only your career but also your supervisor's, ethically and legally. Of course, you should continue your liability coverage after you graduate and get licensed, and throughout the rest of your professional career. If you are sued, immediately notify your liability insurance carrier and your agency. Both parties will provide attorneys to consult with and advise on how to move forward.

If you practice long enough, you will most likely eventually receive a subpoena and/or be part of a client's court case in some capacity. A subpoena is most often issued by a court/judge (sometimes attorney), which requests either your testimony ("subpoena ad testificandum") or your records or related documents ("subpoena duces tecum"). A subpoena does not necessarily mean you are in trouble. Rather, you might be asked to testify, provide a deposition, be an expert witness, serve as a competency examiner, or produce documents related to the case. Thus, you may, or may not, be the counselor of the client in court. When you are served a subpoena, you should accept and respond to this legal document. After accepting, consult with your attorney and inform your supervisor and agency. Your agency needs to know and may have its own protocol and attorneys. It is generally advised that you do not talk to anyone about the subpoena except your attorney, supervisor, and representatives of your agency. How to respond to different subpoena requests (e.g., what records to share vs. privileged communication or how to answer deposition questions) is well beyond the scope of this text and best answered by an attorney who knows the specifics of the case. Ultimately, you cannot ignore a subpoena. That is illegal, and you will be held in contempt of court (i.e., a bench warrant for your arrest). This is very bad.

Assuring Ethical Practice for Mental Health Counselors

The ACA and AMHCA codes of ethics are very thorough in covering all facets related to the profession of counseling. Table 2.1 provides a list of ethics codes that are generally of most interest to mental health counselors

Table 2.1   Ethics Codes of Interest to Mental Health Counselors

Ethics Code	Brief Description	Potential Ethical Concerns
Informed Consent	• Clients have the right to be informed about their rights and responsibilities of their therapy • Clients have self-determination and autonomy to make their own decisions	• It is more than just signing forms; not being clear and up-front about informed consent can damage trust and disempower clients
Confidentiality (subsumed under informed consent)	• What clients disclose to you in counseling must be kept private with a few limitations and exceptions (e.g., as a mandated reporter you have a duty to warn and protect from harm to self or others) • Clients are in charge of their confidentiality; information is generally released only upon their request (unless mandated by law)	• Not being clear about limitations and exceptions to confidentiality (e.g., as a mandated reporter) can damage trust and disempower clients • Privacy concerns with use of modern technology (e.g., electronically stored client information, email, social media, online counseling)
Assessment and Diagnosis	• Assessment should be an ongoing process throughout counseling and is important for case formulation, diagnosis, treatment plans, and interventions • A formal diagnosis is often required by managed care for reimbursement of counseling • Clients should be collaboratively involved and fully informed of the assessments used, and interpretation/conclusions need to be clearly communicated	• Certain assessments and the diagnostic approach may not fully take into consideration cultural factors, which can result in unintentional biases of clients • Must use assessments only after appropriate training and competency • The diagnostic approach is vulnerable to pathologizing clients, especially those that come from oppressed and/or diverse groups • Primarily giving a client a formal diagnosis (possibly exaggerating or minimizing diagnosis) for managed care reimbursement purposes

Competence and Malpractice	• Competence means having the training and skills to effectively and appropriately treat clients in a specific area of practice • Malpractice includes intentional misconduct, unintentional misconduct, or incompetency • The welfare of clients should be put first, including being treated with dignity and respect • If not competent with presenting issues of a client, counselors should refer out to other mental health professionals • Counselors should continually monitor/assess the effectiveness of their counseling with clients • Only empirically supported interventions should be used; or client informed if research on intervention is not robust	• Practicing outside one's scope of competence (i.e., not trained and/or not receiving supervision) • Practicing when impaired (e.g., substance abuse, significant mental health distress, burnout) • Incompetence can result in harming clients, even if not intended; this can result in malpractice lawsuits
Multiple Relationships	• A multiple relationship is when a counselor has two or more concurrent roles or sequential roles with a client • Counselors are advised to minimize having multiple relationships with clients, but it is recognized that some relationships can be unavoidable/part of daily lives • Sexual or romantic relationships with clients are strictly prohibited (includes their romantic partners and family members); or engaging in counseling with a past sexual or romantic partner • It is strongly recommended to avoid any financial/business or personal relationships with clients	• Multiple relationships with clients can diminish professional judgment and increase risk of harming clients • Sexual or romantic relationships with clients are exploitive and almost always cause significant emotional distress; can result in civil or criminal charges • Engaging in financial or business relationships with clients can be exploitive and also compromise trust and objectivity; can result in civil charges

(continued)

	• If a dual relationship cannot be avoided (e.g., elementary teacher at your child's school) or may be potentially beneficial (e.g., attending a graduation), counselors should utilize an accepted ethical decision-making model while taking appropriate precautionary steps including supervision, consultation, informed consent, and documentation • Counselors should also have a social media policy that limits or fully restricts virtual relationships (e.g., social media friend request)	• Entering an unavoidable or potentially beneficial dual relationship without proper planning, supervision, and documentation can put counselors at professional risk and clients at risk of harm
Termination and Abandonment	• Termination can occur when clients have met their treatment goals and/or are no longer benefiting from counseling; this includes a process that happens over time and a mutual agreement to discontinue counseling • Counselors may also decide to discontinue treatment if they believe counseling is harming the client, the client is no longer paying for counseling, or if threats of harm have been made to counselors • If necessary, efforts should be made to refer the client to another mental health professional to continue providing counseling services (e.g., an expert in a particular mental health area)	• Abandonment is when counselors inappropriately end counseling, including not meeting the client's needs • Key factors that contribute to charges of abandonment include not giving the client "adequate notice" of ending counseling and "ample opportunity" to find a new counselor; counselors should help find multiple referrals • Not being honest and clear with reasons for terminating can result in further emotional distress

working with clients. This list includes a brief definition of each ethics code and potential ethical concerns. Because these codes are largely associated with client care, they are often associated with ethical dilemmas and decision-making. You should always use the ACA and/or AMHCA codes of ethics (and relevant state codes of ethics) as your primary guides for making ethical decisions. Although this table is by no means exhaustive, it can be helpful as a quick reference to orient yourself to a basic understanding of what is professionally expected of mental health counselors.

Reflection Questions 2.3: Reviewing Ethics Codes of Interest to Mental Health Counselors

- What are your general thoughts based on all the noted potential ethical concerns? Are there any ethics codes that may be more challenging for you to uphold than others? Why may this be the case?
- Do you have any other ethical concerns beyond the noted ethics codes? Is there an ethics code not addressed that you think should be there? Do you have any other concerns working with clients that may not necessarily be part of an ethics code?
- From a broad perspective of practice, what can you do to avoid the noted potential ethical concerns from occurring?

Activity 2.2: Ethical Dilemmas and Decisions

In a small group of peers, review the following brief scenarios below based on Table 2.1. First, decide if there is a possible ethical dilemma or concern. Then, discuss possible options from an ethical decision perspective (you can also review the Corey et al. [2019] ethical decision-making model discussed earlier).

- Joe runs his own private practice with private pay-only clients (i.e., does not bill through health insurance) and has no other employees (just himself). He values his clients' privacy and never shares any of their personal information with anyone. He only uses electronic record keeping (i.e., no paper) that he keeps on his laptop. He feels confident that his clients' information is secure on his laptop because he has a strong password. Is Joe's clients' information confidentiality secure or do you have some concerns? If you have some concerns, what can he do?
- Jill is a recently licensed therapist who works at a local outpatient agency. Most of her counseling experience is with children and adolescents struggling with depression and oppositional/defiant behaviors. She recently completed an intake for a teenage girl with a trauma history of physical abuse, resulting in what appears to be a diagnosis of PTSD. Jill consulted with her agency supervisor, Susan, on how to move forward. Susan encouraged Jill to keep the case, as this would be good experience for her. Susan has much experience in working

with adolescents and trauma and offered to provide additional supervision support. Is it appropriate for Jill to continue treating her trauma client or do you have some concerns? If you have some concerns, what can she do?

- Josh is seeing a client with mild depressive symptoms due to a major life transition, resulting in a diagnosis of adjustment disorder with depressed mood. The client's health insurance provider allowed for only six sessions. After the fourth session, Josh realized that he will need more than the remaining two sessions to appropriately treat his client. Josh is thinking about changing his client's diagnosis to major depressive disorder because his insurance will allow for more than two sessions. Josh's client is technically two diagnostic symptoms short of having major depressive disorder, but Josh believes this is the right choice in order to provide the care his client needs. Would it be okay for Josh to change his client's diagnosis to have more sessions, or do you have some concerns? If you have some concerns, what can he do?

- Jackie has a client with whom she has good rapport and who has made great progress in therapy. Jackie is looking to update her private practice's website, and it just so happens that her client has expertise in this area. Jackie's client offered to help Jackie update her website for a discounted fee. Jackie initially hesitated because she is still her client. However, Jackie later agreed to follow through with her client's offer, but only after their counseling relationship is over. Would it be okay for Jackie's client to update her website after counseling is complete, or do you have some concerns? If you have some concerns, what can she do?

One way to protect against ethical problems is to proactively behave in a manner that avoids conflicts with specific ethics codes. In other words, know the codes of ethics and do not do anything unethical! This is called risk management. However, worrying too much about potential ethical dilemmas is not ideal professional practice. Rather, instead of worrying about how one can get in trouble, it is best to ask oneself, "Am I being the best counselor I can be?" Many ethical dilemmas result in counselors making "small steps" over time toward crossing professional boundaries. Each small step may individually not get noticed but can accumulate into a giant leap. This shift in professional boundaries is often not noticed until it is too late. This often results out of ignorance of particular codes of ethics and/or trying to handle a situation independently that eventually spirals out of control. Ignorance is not a valid reason for behaving unethically. Table 2.2 highlights best ethical practices for counselors in order to avoid making those small steps toward unethical behavior.

Table 2.2   Best Ethical Practices for Mental Health Counselors

What You Should Know	What You Should Consider
Upfront and Clear about Informed Consent	• Provide clients with informed consent at the very beginning of the counseling relationship • Be very clear about limits of confidentiality, including mandatory reporting • Be clear about billing practices, including disclosing information with managed care
Protect Confidentiality	• Information should only be disclosed with client's permission; unless required by law • Even when information is disclosed, only the minimum information necessary to provide appropriate services should be provided • Every effort should be made to secure confidential information (paper or electronic form)
Understand Multiple Relationships	• Not all multiple relationships are avoidable, but consider whose needs are being met. If it is the counselor's, it is best to avoid the multiple relationships and/or consult • Counselors should consider their power differential, loss of objectivity, and possible exploitation
Thorough Documentation Is Best	• What to document is extensive, but some areas can be overlooked: relevant history for diagnosis, release of information, consultation, treatments/interventions considered and rejected, consent to audiotape or videotape, telephone/email communication, out-of-office contact, attempts to follow up with clients who no-show, supervision feedback after a significant counseling event (e.g., client reported suicidal ideation or explicit flirtation)
Accurate and Truthful Billing	• Be clear with clients from the beginning of counseling how billing works and possible necessary disclosures with managed care • Only bill for the services actually provided (e.g., do not bill for couple therapy when individual therapy is provided or do not bill managed care for a missed appointment) • Accurately identify the dates counseling was actually provided • Regardless of intentions, do not provide an exaggerated or minimized diagnosis • Medical model must be followed for diagnosis, regardless of beliefs; it is illegal not to do so

(continued)

Caution with Self-Disclosure	• Self-disclosure can be an effective treatment technique, but sharing too much information and/or too personal information can harm the counseling relationship and possibly increase client distress • Must consider: is what is being disclosed serving the needs of the counselor or the needs of the client; how does the disclosure help the client's well-being; is the information being disclosed appropriate based on the client's well-being/presenting concerns? • Sharing too much personal information may give a false impression that the counselor has relationship interests beyond/outside of counseling
Caution with Social Media	• It is best to have a clear policy about use of social media, which should at least include not "friending" or "following" (or any other related terminology) each other • Virtual/online relationships should be avoided just like face-to-face relationships outside of counseling; multiple relationships ethics also applies here • Be sure that your own social media content is appropriate and professional, including no available contact information (personal phone number, place of residence) and appropriate private settings; clients do search for content about counselors online • A LinkedIn account is a good way to provide professional information online, and a professional website can be a good source, especially if in private practice
Only Practice in Area of Expertise	• Being well-intentioned, but not realizing when going beyond area of competence can harm clients (e.g., not reduce distress or worsen distress) • Only use interventions after receiving extensive training by qualified experts • Need to keep up with current literature and continue training, rather than relying on the "same old" interventions and assessments over time • This can include modality of therapy (e.g., individual, couple, family, group) and population (e.g., children, adolescents, young adults, middle-age adults, older adults) • If outside realm of competence, supervision and/or consultation may be adequate

Utilize Evidence-Based Practices	• Conceptualize client's problems and distress with an empirically sound theoretical model • Whenever possible, treatment goals and interventions should be supported by robust research (efficacy and effectiveness) • Using evidence-based practices does not mean abandoning your therapeutic style or ignoring client/environmental factors • Utilizing and documenting evidence-based practices provides clients the best opportunity for competent care while minimizing professional risk

Reflection Questions 2.4: Reviewing Best Ethical Practices for Mental Health Counselors

- Are there any best ethical practices that could be personally challenging for you, perhaps with particular client populations? Why may this be the case? What can you do to avoid possible unethical behavior?
- Can you think of any other best ethical practices not noted? What can be done to avoid unethical behavior for these additional best ethical practices?
- What parts of the noted best ethical practices can you envision where a counselor could be vulnerable to making small steps over time to crossing professional boundaries and behaving unethically? What is it about these noted best ethical practices that makes counselors more vulnerable than others?

REFERENCES

American Counseling Association. (2014). *ACA code of ethics*. Author.

American Mental Health Counselors Association. (2020). *AMHCA code of ethics*. Author.

American Mental Health Counselors Association. (2019). AMHCA and ACA separate associations. Retrieved August 15, 2019, from http://www.amhca.org/blogs/howard-goodman/2019/04/26/amhca-and-aca-separate-associations

Auxier, C. R., Hughes, F. R., & Kline, W. B. (2003). Identity development in counselors-in-training. *Counselor Education and Development, 43*, 25–38. https://doi.org/10.1002/j.1556-6978.2003.tb01827.x

Beauchamp, T. L, & Childress, J. F. (2012). *Principles of biomedical ethics* (7th ed.). Oxford University Press.

Corey, G., Corey, M. S., & Corey, C. (2019). *Issues and ethics in the helping professions* (10th ed.). Cengage Learning.

Dollarhide, C. T., & Miller, G. M. (2006). Supervision for preparation and practice of school counselors: Pathways to excellence. Special Section. *Counselor Education and Supervision, 45*, 242–252. https://doi.org/10.1002/j.1556-6978.2006.tb00001.x

Gibson, D. M., Dollarhide, C. T., & Moss, J. M. (2010). Professional identity development: A grounded theory of transformational tasks of new counselors. *Counselor Education and Supervision, 50*, 21–38. https://doi.org/10.1002/j.1556-6978.2010.tb00106.x

Granello, D. H., & Young, M. E. (2019). *Counseling today: Foundations of professional identity* (2nd ed.). Pearson.

Kitchener, K. S. (1984). Intuition, critical evaluation and ethical principles. *The Counseling Psychologist, 12*(3), 43–55. https://doi.org/10.1177/0011000084123005

Lloyd-Hazlett, J., & Foster, V. A. (2016). Student counselors' moral, intellectual, and professional ethical identity development. *Counseling and Values, 62*, 90–105. https://doi.org/10.1002/cvj.12051

Meara, N. M., Schmidt, L. D., & Day, J. D. (1996). Principles and virtues: A foundation for ethical decisions, policies, and character. *The Counseling Psychologist, 24*, 4–77. https://doi.org/10.1177/0011000096241002

Mellin, E. A., Hunt, B., & Nichols, L. M. (2011). Counselor professional identity: Findings and implications for counseling and interprofessional collaboration. *Journal of Counseling and Development, 89*, 140–147. https://doi.org/10.1002/j.1556-6678.2011.tb00071.x

Myers, J. E., Sweeney, T. J., & White, V. E. (2002). Advocacy for counseling and counselors: A professional imperative. *Journal of Counseling and Development, 80*, 394–402. https://doi.org/10.1002/j.1556-6678.2002.tb00205.x

Myers, J. E., Sweeney, T. J., & Witmer, J. M. (2000). The wheel of wellness counseling for wellness: A holistic model for treatment planning. *Journal of Counseling and Development, 78*, 251–266. https://doi.org/10.1002/j.1556-6676.2000.tb01906.x

O'Byrne, K., & Rosenberg, J. I. (1998). The practice of supervision: A sociocultural perspective. *Counselor Education and Supervision, 38*, 34–42. https://doi.org/10.1002/j.1556-6978.1998.tb00555.x

Seiler, G., & Messina, J. J. (1979). Toward professional identity: The dimension of mental health counseling in perspective. *American Mental Health Counselors Journal, 1*, 3–8.

ADDITIONAL RESOURCES

American Counseling Association (ACA) website: www.counseling.org

American Mental Health Counselors Association (AMHCA) website: www.amhca.org

Council for Accreditation of Counseling and Related Educational Programs (CACREP) website: www.cacrep.org

Dong, S., Miles, L., Abell, N., & Martinez, J. (2018). Development of professional identity for counseling professionals: A mindfulness-based perspective. *International Journal for the Advancement of Counselling, 40*, 469–480. https://doi.org/10.1007/s10447-018-9338-y

Masters in Psychology and Counseling Accreditation Council (MPCAC) website: www.mpcacaccreditation.org

Ronnestad, M. H., & Skovholt T. (2012). *The developing practitioner: Growth and stagnation of therapists and counselors*. Routledge.

Ronnestad, M. H., Orlinsky, D. E., Schroder, T. A., Skovholt, T. M., & Willutzki, U. (2018). The professional development of counsellors and psychotherapists: Implications and empirical studies for supervision, training and practice. *Counseling and Psychotherapy Research, 19*, 214–230. https://doi.org/10.1002/capr.12198

Woo, H., Lu, J., Harris, C., & Cauley, B. (2017). Professional identity development in counseling professionals. *Counseling Outcome Research and Evaluation, 8*, 15–30. https://doi.org/10.1080/03054985.2017.1297184

3

Education and Licensure Requirements

■ ■ ■

It takes considerable time and effort to become a licensed mental health counselor. In most states, the earliest you can get your license from the time you enter graduate school is four years. Many graduate programs will take two years to finish as a full-time student. Thereafter, you will need a minimum of two years of postgraduate supervised counseling experience before you can submit your application for licensure. You will also need to pass a specific licensure exam before submitting your application. Of course, this is all after receiving your bachelor's degree. In short, becoming a licensed mental health counselor is a serious commitment in both time and money. However, if it is something you are passionate about, being a licensed practitioner provides many career opportunities, often with much flexibility.

Knowing the amount of time, commitment, and money that it takes from entering graduate school to getting licensed, the last thing you want is the added stress of scrambling toward the end of your journey, making sure (or hoping!) that you can get licensed. The earlier you plan ahead and know the required upcoming steps, the less stressed you will be on your journey to getting licensed. For example, you do not want to enter a graduate program that does not lead to licensure in your desired state (e.g., not enough credit hours or inappropriate curriculum content); or, not receive appropriate supervised postgraduate counseling hours (e.g., supervisor not licensed or not appropriate license). These are just two of many examples of the types of mistakes that can be made while working toward licensure. Some mistakes can be quickly remedied (e.g., forgotten signature on a licensure application), while others can set you back years (e.g., graduate program does not lead to licensure). With that said, if you prepare in advance for the state you want to get licensed in, the process can be relatively smooth with minimal confusion.

This chapter follows the most common sequence of education and experience requirements for licensure. Although each state has its own specific requirements for licensure, most states are similar in their requirements with occasional slight variations. First, key factors to consider when selecting a graduate program in counseling, ranging from quality of course content to practicum and internship training opportunities, are discussed. Next, your experience postgraduation, namely obtaining postgraduate counseling experience, is reviewed. Thereafter, credentialing and licensure, including the two most common licensure exams and other required exams by some states (e.g., jurisprudence exam), are addressed. Next, key components of a licensure application, including common mistakes to avoid, are reviewed. Finally, license portability across states is addressed. Appendix 1 provides an extensive list of all fifty states and key requirements for licensure: state licensure website, licensure title, graduate program credit hours, accreditation, counseling experience requirements, and required licensure exam(s). It is highly suggested that you refer to this list when researching any states in which you plan to obtain licensure as you read through each section of this chapter.

GRADUATE DEGREE IN COUNSELING

One obvious first step in becoming a licensed mental health counselor is getting the appropriate education in a graduate counseling program. Most counseling graduate programs are moderately competitive. Typically, most programs expect at least a 3.0 GPA (some may require 2.75 and others 3.25), three letters of recommendations from professors and/or other professionals who have supervised any work you have done in the field, a personal statement specific to the program's expectations, and a résumé. It is preferable to highlight in your résumé any service experience (e.g., undergrad internship, summer volunteer work) and any leadership experience (e.g., vice president of the psychology club). Some programs may also require Graduate Record Examination (GRE) scores and/or GRE Psychology scores. As part of the application process, you may be required to participate in individual and/or group interviews. Programs typically use these interviews as an opportunity to assess your interpersonal skills, emotional intelligence, problem-solving ability, and overall potential for success in graduate school. Of course, interviews are also a great opportunity for you to learn more about the program, especially through interactions with faculty and current students.

One common inaccurate assumption is that one must major in psychology in order to apply for a graduate program in counseling. In most cases, you do not need a major in psychology, but in some cases you may need to meet a minimum number of psychology courses; a few programs will note specific psychology courses. Other common bachelor's degrees besides psychology include sociology, human services, special education, child/family studies, and criminal justice. Other less common, but still often acceptable, bachelor's degrees include teacher education, English, political science, business, communications, and biology. Remember, these lists are just examples, students can have a variety of backgrounds as long as they meet the program's application requirements.

Just as graduate programs in counseling will be assessing your "fit" for their program, you will be assessing their ability to meet your academic and professional (i.e., licensure) needs. You will be a graduate student for approximately two or three years; it will take a considerable amount of your time and money. You want your experience to be pleasant while you are developing competency in counseling skills that will eventually be used to help others. Stated differently, make sure you choose a program that fully prepares you to be a competent licensed mental health counselor. The following addresses some of the most important components of training that you should consider when selecting, and enrolled in, a graduate program in counseling.

General Graduate Program Qualities for Consideration

There are a few important qualities to consider when selecting graduate programs in counseling. Some of these qualities are explicit, while others are not as obvious. Thus, the following discussion attempts to highlight some of the more significant nuances and strategies that should be considered when selecting a graduate program in counseling.

Pragmatically, what matters most about the graduate program you attend is that it will lead to licensure as a professional mental health counselor in the state in which you want to practice. Many times, students attend graduate programs in the state they want to get licensed in, but this is not always the case. (Portability of licensure will be discussed at the end of this chapter.) Thus, the name of the actual program and degree offered is less important than the actual training that leads to licensure. Common examples of names of graduate programs in counseling include mental health counseling, clinical mental health counseling, clinical community mental health, counseling psychology, clinical psychology, clinical-counseling psychology, applied psychology, school counseling, and counselor education. (It is important to note here that use of the term "psychology" in program titles does not mean graduating students will be psychologists. The term psychologist is reserved for those that graduate with a doctoral degree [e.g., Ph.D. or Psy.D.].) There most likely will be some differences in curriculum based on program name/degree (e.g., clinical-counseling psychology program vs. counselor education), but there will be more similarities with regard to required core content for state requirements for licensure. The differences often come down to background in core faculty and theoretical orientation of the program. These differences may still matter to you if you are looking for a particular focus in training.

Quality programs should be clear that their degrees lead to licensure in their respective states. This includes content on their website, program handbook/brochures, and direct conversation with faculty. Keep in mind, no program can promise that you will get licensed. Rather, programs can tout that their curriculum and training put you in the position to get licensed. You are the one responsible for obtaining appropriate postgraduate training, passing the licensing exam, and appropriately submitting your application materials.

Ultimately, it is up to you to do your own research up front to ensure that the program matches state requirements for licensing. If you are not sure (and even if you are sure), it is best to speak with the program director and other faculty that teach in the program. If there is still any ambiguity, including incomplete answers to your questions, it may be best to avoid the program. Keep in mind that most programs may not be able to answer licensing questions outside their respective state. To be fair, do not expect programs to focus on state licensing standards for all fifty states. It would not be possible for any program to meet this expectation. Thus, it will be up to you to take the extra steps to research any states in which you think you may eventually want to receive licensure. In many cases, you might only have to take an extra class or two, or need some additional practicum/internship hours. Most programs are flexible to let you make these minor modifications if you inform them ahead of time.

Beyond licensure, it is strongly suggested that you ask around the community and current/former students about the reputation of the program. For example, are students satisfied with the program? What are student–faculty and student–student relationships like? Are students graduating? Are they graduating with clinical/counseling skills? Are they getting placements for their practicum/internships? Are they getting jobs in reputable agencies after graduation? Are graduates prepared/passing the licensure exam? Are they getting licensed? If you ask, most programs will let you openly ask faculty these questions. More importantly, it is helpful to talk to any current students and recent graduates employed in the field. Sometimes programs will have student and alumni representatives readily available to answer your questions. Programs may even provide contact information of local mental health agencies who can speak to current program trainee and employee competency.

Program Curriculum: Credit Hours and Course Content
You will need to know the total number of required total degree semester hours (i.e., credits) for the program you enroll in and how many are

required for the states you want to pursue licensure in. Most states now require 60 credits, with some that are 48 credits; a few do not provide a minimum number of credits. Over time, the number of total degree semester hours can change by increasing, but not decreasing. The most common trend over the past decade has been states with 48 credits increasing to 60 credits and states with no minimum to 48 or 60 credits. It is not expected that any state will go above 60 credits in the foreseeable future.

Appropriate total credits is a prerequisite for licensure. In some states, you must receive all your credits from the same program for licensure. In other words, you cannot take additional credits after graduation. In this case (e.g., even if you received 59 credits out of 60 required), you would need to enroll in another program that provides the appropriate number of credits (i.e., start over from the beginning). In other states, you might be able to get most of your credits from one program (e.g., 48 credits) and then later take additional courses to meet the required total credits for state licensure (e.g., take an additional 12 credits for a total of 60 credits). However, this situation is not ideal because it may delay the time it takes to obtain licensure. For example, typically your postgraduate counseling hours start after you graduate. However, some states will not count postgraduate counseling hours until after the full total of credits is met (e.g., after 60 credits have been obtained). To avoid all this confusion, it is wisest to simply enroll in a program that provides all the necessary credits for licensure.

In addition to required credits, all states require coverage of "core content areas." What this means is that not just number of credits is important. The specific content of the courses that make up the total credits is also relevant for state licensure requirements. For example, Massachusetts requires 60 credits and has 10 core content areas: counseling theory, human growth and development, psychopathology, social and cultural foundations, clinical skills, group work, special treatment issues, appraisal, research and evaluation, and professional orientation. Many states have very similar core content areas, but there can still be minor variations. Most programs openly identify all their required courses, including a description, and how each course aligns with the state core content areas. Programs that follow state licensure requirements purposely arrange their course names and content to ensure that the state core content areas are met. These state core content areas are not developed randomly. Experts in the field determine these core content areas based on the premise that they are necessary for the development of a competent mental health counselor. Also, much of the content should be helpful in passing the required state licensing exam. Overall, be sure the programs you apply to meet not only the total degree semester hour requirements but also the core content areas as well. Be leery of programs that are not clear in how their course content matches state licensure requirements. Just having the total credits is not enough. It is probably best to avoid any programs that cannot confidently identify how each of their courses matches the specific required state core content areas.

A final comment should be made here about total credits and core content areas. You may find yourself enrolled in a program that meets its state total course credits and content requirements for licensure, but you are considering pursuing licensure in another state. First, as soon as possible, check the licensure requirements of any state you may want to get licensed in. Second, compare the total credits and content of your program with these states. You may notice a few slight variations, but all is most likely not lost. If you talk to the program director early in your matriculation, you may be able to negotiate taking extra courses while in the program. For example, you may notice that a specific course is not required in the state the program is in, but required in another state in which you want to get licensure. You might be able to do an independent study for that particular course. Another example is simply not having enough credits. Perhaps the program you are in requires only 48 total credits but you need 60 credits. There is a good chance that the program would let you take additional courses (in this case four), assuming that there are additional courses available to take (or you can do an independent study).

You may also notice that some programs have theoretical orientations (e.g., cognitive-behavioral therapy [CBT]) or specializations (e.g., child and family studies). This may be something of interest to you if you would like to specialize in a particular evidence-based theoretical approach or know what population(s) you would like to work with. Training in particular approaches can result in future certifications (see "Certification" section). Although such certifications can be beneficial to your career, you still need to make sure that the program you attend leads to licensure. In most circumstances, a certification will not have much value, or not be possible to obtain, without being licensed to practice.

Program Accreditation

Another factor that may be relevant to licensure in specific states is accreditation. There are currently two major accreditation agencies: Council for Accreditation of Counseling and Related Education Programs (CACREP) and Masters in Psychology and Counseling Accreditation Council (MPCAC). There are currently a few states that require CACREP accreditation. This is largely due to strong lobbying efforts by CACREP and its affiliation with the American Counseling Association (ACA). Some have raised concerns about this requirement because it excludes many strong programs in counseling/psychology that follow evidence-based practice (Campbell et al., 2018; Hughes & Diaz-Granados, 2018). MPCAC has taken an inclusionary approach by providing accreditation that meets its high evidence-based standards but not at the expense of those not accredited by MPCAC. A key quote from MPCAC's (2021) "Frequently Asked Questions" web page states the following:

> Several fields (such as nursing, business, psychology) offer multiple pathways to achieve core competencies and therefore credentialing; the practice of counseling and psychological services at the master's level is no exception. Most fields, particularly those in the health care arena, recognize the added value of diversity in training, and the danger of group-think when such diversity is lacking. Science-based principles and practices develop most freely in an environment that fosters interdisciplinary work and steers away from rigid intellectual silos. Therefore, the existence of multiple accrediting bodies promotes the richness of a field and consequently the public good.

Over time, more states will most likely begin requiring accreditation by either CACREP, MPCAC, or both. There is currently a movement to have states accept either CACREP or MPCAC instead of one or the other—"counseling for all" (Alliance for Professional Counselors, 2021). Also, the American Psychological Association (APA) is in the early stages of considering accrediting/licensing master's level counselors (without using the title "psychologist"), perhaps with MPCAC (Buckman et al., 2018; Hughes & Diaz-Granados, 2018). Hopefully, a more inclusionary approach will be taken to recognize diversity in programs for state licensure, as long as core state curriculum content is met through evidence-based training. Nevertheless, be sure that the program you enroll in provides the necessary accreditation for the state you want to practice in.

Program Practicum and Internship Training Opportunities
One of the key defining steps of your graduate training is obtaining field experience where you get to formally apply your newly acquired counseling skills. This is a significant step in your professional development in the field, including working face-to-face with clients while receiving supervision from licensed mental health professionals. Typically, most programs have you begin with your practicum after approximately one year of coursework and include approximately 100–200 hours of experience. In some programs/states the practicum consists of a small classroom setting where you get to practice your counseling skills by role-playing with your peers while being supervised by your instructor. In other programs/states the practicum is an actual field placement with a local mental health agency where you eventually get the opportunity to provide face-to-face counseling with clients under the supervision of a licensed mental health professional. Notice here that you will need a licensed supervisor for both your practicum and internship.

If not, your counseling hours will not count toward licensure. Also, keep in mind that some states require a ratio of client hours to supervision hours (e.g., 16:1—1 hour of supervision for every 16 client hours). Additionally, if you would like to receive training through a particular theoretical orientation and/or population, make sure your supervisor has these experiences. This is the first opportunity to get "the feel" for what it is like (at least in part) to be a mental health counselor, and you want to make the best of it. (Chapter 5 focuses on obtaining a job, but it can also be helpful for finding a quality practicum/internship placement and appropriate supervisor.) Finally, your program should also remind you that before you begin to see clients, you will need to obtain liability insurance. The two most common options for counselors include CPH & Associates (endorsed by American Mental Health Counselors Association [AMHCA]) and Healthcare Providers Service Organization (endorsed by ACA). As noted in Chapter 2, although you fall under your supervisor's license (who should also have liability insurance), obtaining liability insurance is a must to protect your assets in case of an act of negligence.

After you complete your practicum, you typically begin your internship for the next two semesters, which includes approximately 600–800 hours of experience. If you did not have face-to-face client hours during your practicum, you will definitely be doing this in your internship. The mental health agency you intern at may be the same as your practicum or a different agency. During your internship you will obviously still receive supervision by a licensed mental health professional, but you will most likely have more client hours and additional duties than you did in your practicum experience. For example, you might be doing client intakes, group therapy, crisis management, participating in treatment teams, and attending meetings with outside providers. Also, expectations of counseling skills will begin to increase over time. This does not mean your supervisors or program will expect you to be an expert in counseling. Rather, there should be some gradual growth in counseling skills and overall professional development from the beginning of your practicum to the end of your internship (approximately one year of field training).

Many students view their practicum and internship experiences as meaningful milestones in their professional development. Taking theory and counseling techniques learned in class, applying them to "real clients" with quality supervision, and noticing clients' well-being improve over time can be an exhilarating experience. These experiences typically confirm one's desire to be a counselor, while also helping a few realize that counseling may not be the profession for them. Your development as a professional counselor has many components beyond good counseling skills: getting along well with colleagues, being able to work independently but know when to seek supervision, practicing ethically, completing paperwork well and on time, developing appropriate treatment goals and interventions, being able to problem-solve, appropriately coping while under stress, and taking feedback well from colleagues. Your practicum and internship experience is the first time you get to develop these skills within the context of a mental health counselor while being supervised by other professionals. Starting off in the right direction is important, as this will be the first major milestone in your professional development. Your next step after graduation will be your first job as a mental health counselor. Your practicum or internship placement may be your potential employer or at the very least your supervisors will be references for future jobs. Overall, your practicum and internship experience can be a stepping-stone for future job opportunities and social networking. You can now begin establishing your professional reputation in the community. Make the best of these experiences!

Finally, similar to course content and credit hours, be sure that your practicum and internship provide the necessary hours for the state you want to get licensed in. You may have noticed earlier that a range of 100–200 hours for practicum and 600–800 hours for internship was provided. This is the average required hours based on state licensure requirements, but this can vary across individual states. Having more hours than you need is not a problem. However, if you will not get enough hours based on program/state requirements, then it is best to talk to your program director and practicum/internship agency supervisor in advance. Requesting additional hours is usually not a problem for most agencies unless they have specific restrictions in place related to training (e.g., not enough clients; supervision availability). It is best to get your required practicum/internship hours while matriculated in your program, before graduating. After graduating, it can sometimes be difficult to obtain the additional 100–200 hours. Many programs will not let you do a partial practicum or internship. You will most likely have to do another semester (or two) of training, which can delay getting licensed and obtaining full-time employment.

Program Capstone Experience

Most graduate programs will have a final capstone experience to demonstrate your overall knowledge of counseling based on course content and, hopefully, integration of your counseling skills. Common examples are a thesis, a comprehensive exam, or an oral exam. A thesis is typically more research based, but there are ways to include integration of counseling skills. A comprehensive exam can be developed by the program and include both theoretical and counseling skills, or an external exam can be used, such as the National Counselor Examination (NCE; discussed in detail in the "Licensure Exams" section), which is more course content based. Oral exams are typically integrative of both course content and counseling skills (e.g., identify theories and present a case with a treatment plan and interventions supported by research). Regardless of the means of evaluation, the goal is for you to demonstrate enough competency to warrant a graduate degree and be ready to be at least a prelicensed mental health counselor. Do not take your program's capstone experience lightly. Graduating with your degree is often dependent on passing.

Reflection Questions 3.1: Graduate Program Experience

- Besides having a curriculum and training opportunities that prepare you for licensure, what are other important qualities to look for in a graduate program?
- How important to you is program theoretical orientation and/or specializations?
- What type of setting/population would you like to work with during your practicum and internship?
- What are important qualities to look for in a practicum/internship agency?
- What are important qualities to look for in your practicum/internship supervisor?

Activity 3.1: Research State Licensure Requirements

Take some time to consider what state(s) you plan on getting licensed in. You may immediately already know the state(s). In other cases, you may have to consider your future plans (e.g., family, personal desire to live in a particular location) to determine the state(s). You may also not be completely sure, but have a few ideas; thus, you may need to consider multiple states. Once you have a general sense of what state(s) you would like to be licensed in, refer to Appendix 1, which provides a list of all fifty states for licensure. Then, review the key requirements (i.e., licensure title, graduate program credit hours, accreditation, counseling experience requirements, and required licensure exam[s]) and review the state licensure website(s). It is best to know as much information as possible before applying for licensure a few years down the road. Consider the following:

- Identify any states you are sure you will apply for licensure.
- Identify any states you might apply for licensure.
- Compare the graduate programs you are considering (or currently enrolled in) with state requirements for:
  - Total credit hours and course content (including accreditation, if applicable).

- Total practicum and internship counseling hours, including definition of approved supervisor.
- Total postgraduate counseling hours, including definition of approved supervisor.
- Licensure exam and any other exams (e.g., jurisprudence exam).
- Possibility of different licensure levels and associated requirements.
- If necessary, make a list of the above-noted differences between your current program and the state you want to get licensed in, and then contact the program director as soon as possible to develop a plan.

POSTGRADUATE EXPERIENCE

Graduating with your degree in counseling is a significant professional and life accomplishment. You have already completed many necessary steps required for licensure. However, in most states, you will still need to work full-time for approximately two years (three to four years if part-time) before you can get licensed. The average range of required hours for most states is 2,000–4,000 hours. In some states, there are multiple levels of licensure, including an "initial license" soon after graduation (i.e., technically a pre-licensure) that requires supervision (discussed more in the "Licensure" section). Regardless, you will need to make sure you obtain a job with a mental health agency that allows you to get enough client hours with appropriate supervision. Keep in mind that states vary in their expectation of agency availability of supervisors and payment for supervision. In some states, the agency that employs you will provide supervision on-site at no cost to you. In other states, not all agencies will provide on-site supervision and you may have to search for an available board-approved supervisor and pay for supervision services. Finally, as with your practicum/internship experience, if you have a choice, try to obtain a supervisor that is a good fit for your desired professional development (e.g., population and disorder/problem expertise, evidence-based interventions, theoretical orientation). Also, be sure that your supervisor meets the state's approved supervisor requirements and you receive the appropriate client hours–supervision ratio, or your hours will not count toward licensure.

Although you will still receive constant supervision of your counseling as you did in your practicum/internship, do not expect your overall experience as a professional counselor to be the same (even if you are working at the same agency as your practicum/internship). You are now a paid employee for an agency. Hopefully, you will work for an agency that recognizes where you are in your professional career development. Nevertheless, you will have many responsibilities and will be expected to work more independently than you did in your practicum/internship. You may also find that your supervision will focus less on counseling skills and include many administrative matters as well. Overall, although you are not yet licensed, you are still considered a professional mental health counselor with most of the same expectations and ethical standards as your licensed colleagues.

Your postgraduate experience in many ways can have a strong impact on your career path and professional development. This is your opportunity to learn even more about the "real world" of being a mental health counselor. In other words, not only will you continue to develop your counseling skills, you will also learn more about what goes on behind the scenes with regard to managed care organizations, administrative practices, and working with colleagues from other professions (to name a few). These experiences may challenge and change some of your assumptions about the counseling field, and perhaps how you view humanity. Furthermore, the populations you work with and the settings you work in can put you in a position toward eventually being an expert with a particular population (e.g., adolescents with trauma histories). Of course, your first job does not have to dictate your future career path, but it can at least provide a strong foundation for future employment and promotion opportunities.

Reflection Questions 3.2: Postgraduate Experience

- What do you expect to be different from your practicum/internship compared to your postgraduate counseling experience?
- What are important qualities to look for in your postgraduate supervisor? Are any of these qualities different from what you look for in your practicum/internship supervisor? Explain.
- What are your thoughts and feelings about having most of the same responsibilities as your licensed colleagues early in your career?
- What are your thoughts about considering a population and/or setting to specialize in at this point in your career (i.e., too early or appropriate time?)?

CERTIFICATION

Before discussing licensure, there is also the option to receive certification. Some certifications can be obtained while in graduate school or postgraduate pre-licensure. Certification is a credential from a particular professional organization that provides recognition that a professional has met particular standards of specialized practice (e.g., examinations, training, counseling experience). The organizations that provide these certifications are made up of a body of professional peers who are also experts in that particular specialized practice. A graduate degree typically demonstrates general knowledge of counseling (still very important), whereas a certification signifies a purposeful approach in additional study and counseling experience in a specialized area.

The National Board for Certified Counselors (NBCC) is the largest organization that provides counselors general certification and specialized certifications. The most widely known and obtained certification is the National Certified Counselor (NCC) credential. Being NCC certified means that you have met NBCC's highest training standards. However, beginning in 2022, only individuals from a CACREP-accredited program will be able to obtain the NCC credential. After being NCC certified, you can pursue other specialized certifications offered by the NBCC including a Certified Clinical Mental Health Counselor (CCMHC), a National Certified School Counselor (NCSC), and a Master Addictions Counselor (MAC). The Center for Credentialing and Education (CCE), an affiliate of NBCC, also offers an Approved Clinical Supervisor (ACS) certification.

Specialized training while in graduate school and postgraduate counseling experience can result in other certifications specific to evidence-based approaches and populations served. For example, you can receive a CBT certification from the Academy of Cognitive and Behavioral Therapies and/or the Beck Institute if specific curriculum and counseling training requirements are met. Such certifications from particular organizations not only provide professional identification and document competence in a specialized skill set but also can potentially enhance your practice and professional recognition.

LICENSURE EXAMS

All states require a licensure exam. In some cases, it may be best to take the state licensure exam soon after graduation. In other cases, it may be best to wait until you are close to the required total postgraduate hours. When you take the exam usually depends on the actual exam itself and your personal preference. As stated earlier, the program you received your degree from should prepare you well for the licensure exam. However, many find that their postgraduate experience, including seeing a variety of clients with a variety of presenting problems, also has added much value to their preparation to pass the licensure exam.

The two most common licensure exams are the National Counselor Examination (NCE) and the National Clinical Mental Health Counseling Examination (NCMHCE). Both of these exams are owned and administered by the NBCC. All 50 states accept the NCE and/or NCMHCE as a valid licensure exam. These exams are evaluated twice a year by an exam committee to review recent examinee performance, review and remove potentially problematic items, consider and implement new items for consideration, and review and modify cutoff scores (NBCC, 2021). There are a few states that may accept an alternative exam and/or require a jurisprudence exam. Passing the licensure exam and completing the rest of your application materials will result in you receiving your license and formal title from your respective state.

Two of the most common license titles are licensed mental health counselor (LMHC) and licensed professional counselor (LPC). As briefly touched upon earlier, some states have multiple licensure tiers (up to four!). This is often based on total program credits and/or postgraduate supervised hours. This means some states have a step process where you can receive an initial license soon after graduation (i.e., technically a pre-licensure) while direct supervision is still required and then work your way up to a more independent license as you gain additional postgraduate supervised hours (and possibly take an additional licensure exam). For example, some states allow postgraduate beginning counselors to be titled as "Licensed Associate Counselor" or "Registered Mental Health Counselor Intern" to indicate continued postgraduate supervision. There may be a ceiling on your license level if you do not meet the required program credits for a "higher" licensure level. Depending on the state, you may, or may not, be able to return to graduate school for these additional credits. Ideally, your goal from the beginning of your education and training should always be the highest level of licensure to ensure your ability to practice independently and provide yourself the most career advancement opportunities.

The following provides a review of the most common licensure exams, other exam requirements by some states, and some comments about preparing for licensure exams. Refer to Appendix 1, which identifies the required exams and license titles for each state.

National Counselor Examination

The NCE is the most common exam required for state licensure and is used for national certification. The NCE can also be taken by students advanced in their graduate program for national certification if their program has received NBCC approval (see the "Certification" section discussed earlier). The NCE focuses on the eight CACREP content areas: human growth and development, social and cultural diversity, counseling and helping relationships, group counseling and group work, career counseling, assessment and testing, research and program evaluation, and professional orientation and ethical practice. Skills and abilities are assessed through five work behavior domains: fundamental counseling issues; counseling process;

diagnostic and assessment services; professional practice; and professional development, supervision, and consultation. The NCE is computer-based administered (although paper and pencil in some cases) and consists of 200 multiple-choice questions (i.e., four choices each) to be completed within four hours. Each of the eight content areas has 25 questions (from a larger test bank of items). However, five of the 25 questions are new questions being piloted for potential future use. Thus, there is a total of 160 questions that will count toward the passing cutoff score. Of course, you do not know which of the questions are part of the exam or piloted, so each of the questions should be treated as if they are counted as part of the cutoff score. It is important to note that passing the exam is based only on the examinee's knowledge, not compared to the performance of others (i.e., the cutoff score is criterion based, not norm based). If you do not pass, you can retake the exam once every three months. More information about the NCE can be found at the NBCC website (www.nbcc.org/exams/nce).

National Clinical Mental Health Counseling Examination

The NCMHCE is the second-most common exam required for state licensure. Some states solely require the NCMHCE for licensure, while others require both the NCE and NCMHCE. The NCMHCE is also used for certification as a Certified Clinical Mental Health Counselor. It is important to note that the NBCC (2021) has just completed major revisions to the questions and format of the NCMHCE, which will go into effect in 2022. In order to sit for the NCMHCE, you will have to meet the criteria for a minimally qualified candidate (MQC). To be an MQC for the NCMHCE, you will have to be a graduate (or a "well-advanced graduate student") from a counseling program accredited by CACREP or from a regionally accredited institution (i.e., a non-CACREP program like MPCAC). The counseling program must contain courses in the following content areas: human growth and development theories in counseling, social and cultural foundations in counseling, helping relationships in counseling, group counseling theories and processes, career counseling and lifestyle development, assessment in counseling, research and program evaluation, professional orientation to counseling, and counseling field experience. The NCMHCE is computer-based administered. Although the NCMHCE will now be multiple choice in format, it will still be unique to the NCE in that it will comprise of 12–14 case studies (final number of case studies yet to be determined—pending further field testing) to be completed in 225 minutes. The purpose of the case studies is to assess your ability, as an entry-level counselor, to "identify, analyze, diagnose, and develop plans for treatment of clinical concerns" (NBCC, 2021). Of the 12–14 case studies, two will be unscored and used for statistical analyses for future test forms. Thus, 10–12 case studies will count toward the exam. Similar to the NCE, you do not know which case study is part of the exam or unscored, so all the case studies should be treated as if they are counted as part of the exam.

Each of the case studies is designed to simulate the work of a mental health counselor. Each case study will include one narrative and 10 multiple-choice questions (four options with one correct choice). Bloom's Taxonomy classification framework will be used to assess higher cognitive levels (i.e., comprehension, application, knowledge, evaluation). Within each case study will be three sections: initial intake summary (e.g., demographics, presenting problems, mental status exam, history of condition, family history, work history, current living situation, relationships) and two counseling sessions (e.g., description of current presentation, including progress made from previous sessions). Each section begins with a narrative followed by multiple-choice questions, which are derived from the narrative and measure the following five content domains: professional practice and ethics; intake, assessment, and diagnosis; treatment planning; counseling skills and interventions; and core counseling attributes. Area of clinical focus is the sixth content domain, but there are no multiple-choice questions because this information is provided within the case study itself.

Passing the NCMHCE is based on the total sum of correctly scored items. Each multiple-choice question will be weighted the same (i.e., one point), regardless of case study section or content domain. Statistical analyses (including statistical equating adjustments based on overall difficulty) and NCMHCE Examination Committee review of each question will be used to determine the passing score for each exam. As with the NCE, passing the NCMHCE exam is based only on the examinee's knowledge, not compared to the performance of others (i.e., criterion based, not norm based). If you do not pass, you can retake the exam once every three months. More information about the NCMHCE can be found at the NBCC website (www.nbcc.org/exams/ncmhce).

Other Exams

There are a few states that allow for alternative exams, instead of the NCE or NCMHCE, for licensure. For example, the Certified Rehabilitation Counselor Examination (CRCE) focuses on competency as a rehabilitation counselor. The CRCE is accepted as an alternate licensure exam in many states. Also, the Examination of Clinical Counseling Practice (ECCP) is the original exam used for clinical mental health counseling and is still accepted in Illinois and Minnesota in place of the NCE or the NCMHCE. Overall, simply keep in mind that although all 50 states accept the NCE and/or NCMHCE as a valid licensure exam, there are a few states that have some acceptable alternative options.

Jurisprudence Exam

Over the past 10–20 years, an increasing trend has been licensure boards requiring applicants to pass a jurisprudence exam. Some states require passing the jurisprudence exam to receive initial licensure, while other states require passing the exam for licensure renewal. The purpose of a jurisprudence exam is to assess your knowledge about relevant state laws related to the profession of counseling and the board's rules, including regulations and processes. Examples of content related to state laws include duty to warn when a client threatens to harm another individual (or themselves), limits to client confidentiality, and responding to a subpoena to produce client documents. Examples of content related to the board's rules include background checks for licensure applicants, approved supervisor qualifications, and the process for the board responding to ethical complaints. Obviously, preparing for the content of a jurisprudence exam is state specific, as laws can vary greatly across states.

Other Exam Formats

There are a few select states that use alternative/additional means to obtain licensure. For example, Arkansas requires an oral interview, New Hampshire requires an essay exam, and North Dakota requires a 30-minute taped counseling session. Be sure to check for any unique application requirements in any state where you are considering licensure. You will want to know all requirements as soon as possible to avoid any surprises or confusion.

Counselor Exam Preparation and Practice Opportunities

Sitting for a licensure exam is a challenging and stressful experience for most people. Most counseling students do not think much about licensing exams until soon before they graduate or later into their postgraduate years. This is understandable, considering they are focused on their graduate curriculum and completing their practicum/internship (while possibly even working a part/full-time job!). Because the NCE is more course content based, some counselors prefer to take this exam soon after graduation, or possibly toward the end of their graduate program matriculation if it is allowed (or even required) by their program. On the other hand, many counselors prefer to take the NCMHCE after gaining additional postgraduate counseling hours due to its applied nature (i.e., content is representative of counseling in the field).

Luckily, there are many test preparation materials available for the NCE and NCMHCE, the two exams required (at least one) by all 50 states. It is strongly recommended to start with the preparation guides developed by the NBCC (www.nbcc.org/Exams/ExamPrep). For the NCE, a preparation guide can be purchased for $34.95. This preparation guide includes general information about the exam, a practice test (the only guide with actual retired test items), and tips and strategies. For the NCMHCE, a preparation guide can be purchased for $44.95. This preparation guide includes an explanation on how to take the exam and a five-simulation sample examination, which includes directions for scoring and explanations for each choice (correct and incorrect). Obtaining the NCMHCE preparation guide is highly recommended, considering its case study format and strong emphasis on applied counseling skills.

The NBCC website also provides additional preparation materials from paid advertisers. You can also do your own internet search for alternative preparation materials. These preparation materials are largely online based where you can take practice exams/case studies and obtain supplemental study guides and tips. In some cases, hard-copy materials also are available. Of course, these practice materials come at a price (in some cases a few hundred dollars), largely based on how much content you receive access to and how long you can access the content. Like any study materials, they vary not only in content but also in quality. Be sure to do your own research, including your own initial impressions, online reviews, and talking to counselors who have taken the exams and passed. Counselors who have already passed the exam (especially recently) can not only direct you to helpful resources but also provide you personalized helpful tips.

Many state counseling associations also provide license exam preparation workshops for a fee. These workshops can be extensive in content and strategies, sometimes taking two full days (often a whole weekend). Due to the high cost of some of these workshops (typically over $500), it is recommended to first try the study preparation materials from the NBCC and a reputable preparation website, which are usually cheaper. If you still find yourself not confident in being able to pass the exam, then a workshop may be worth consideration. A workshop is also a good option if you do not pass the exam and still doubt your ability to pass after additional studying.

Some individuals find it helpful to study in groups, both face-to-face and through the Internet. Counselors in your state may have created a study blog or Facebook discussion group. There are even smartphone applications to help study (e.g., search "NCE study"). Regardless of the materials (or workshops) you utilize, be sure to register for a date to take the exam that gives you enough time to study. Then, develop a study plan that includes blocking out days/times for studying. Do not take these exams for granted. No matter how much you think you know the material, you will need to study. These are definitely not exams you pull an "all-nighter" for. Rather, they require much mental focus, including repetition of learning over time. You know how you study best for exams. Just be sure to prepare enough in advance so you can give yourself a good chance of passing. It is your time and money (and career!).

Reflection Questions 3.3: Licensure Exams

- What are your thoughts and feelings about having to take a licensure exam based on a pass/fail to obtain your license?
- What are your thoughts about the different types of licensure exams, including format and type of content?
- Based on your state requirements, type of exams, and personal study habits, when would you like to take your licensure exam (i.e., soon before/after graduation or closer to completion of postgraduate counseling hours)?

Activity 3.2: Search for Study Materials and Study Strategies

Now that you know what exam(s) you need take for licensure, consider what materials and strategies you should utilize to study. First, visit the NBCC website noted earlier (www.nbcc.org/Exams/ExamPrep) to review the exam descriptions and consider purchasing their NCE and/or NCMHCE study guides. These study guides are a good place to start to become more familiar with exam content and style, and they are relatively cheap compared to other study materials. Also review any additional study materials from paid advertisers on the NBCC website. Many of the provided options have a good reputation. Of course, take some time to search the Internet for additional study options. Remember, be sure to check out any reviews for the study materials and also talk to other counselors who have recently studied for the exams to get their perspective. Next, take a look at your state's mental health counselor association and see if they offer any workshops. Finally, consider joining a study blog and/or discussion group and developing a study group with other peers. Overall, plan in advance as much as you can both your study materials and your strategies. It might help to print out the calendar months (or use an Excel spreadsheet) between when you plan to study and the date of your exam. You can then select what dates (and times) you plan to study while also tracking the particular content you studied for and any related notes. Be honest with yourself about the quality and quantity of your study time!

APPLICATION FOR LICENSURE

Each state has its own application requirements, but there are certainly many similarities in the type of content and the overall process. It is a big deal to submit your application for licensure. This is a significant step in your professional development and career. State licensure provides legal permission to independently practice as a professional mental health counselor. It indicates that you are competent to professionally practice. It can potentially open other up career opportunities and promotions, including leadership and administrative positions. It will also most likely mean a pay increase because your license allows you to independently bill health insurance companies (managed care organizations), possibly at a higher rate. You can also consider the option of having an independent/private practice (see Chapter 8).

Keep in mind that licensure boards typically predominately consist of licensed counselors (sometimes from related professions) and exist for the purpose of regulating the practice of a profession. Board members have the responsibility of assuring competency in those that are granted licensure and protecting the public from those who do/would practice unethically, including harm to clients. A licensing board is what makes your profession a profession!

As discussed earlier, in most states you will need an additional two years of postgraduate supervised counseling experience before applying for licensure. As you approach your two years' postgraduate experience you should have already taken your state's required licensing exam. Now is the time to begin putting together all your application materials (if you have not done so already), including supervisor signatures once you reach the postgraduate experience time frame/hours. The following highlights the most common application components along with the most common mistakes to avoid. Remember, it is best to review your state's application materials while you are still matriculated in your graduate program and definitely no later than right after graduation.

Common Licensure Application Components
Like any application, the first few pages consist of basic personal information (e.g., name, mailing address, phone number, email address, date of birth, social security number). You will most likely also be asked to provide a recent head-and-shoulders photograph (i.e., passport photo). There will also be questions if you have ever had disciplinary action taken against you by a licensing board (typically for those who have been licensed in another state) and if you have ever been convicted of a felony or misdemeanor. Relatedly, you will most likely be asked to give permission to have a criminal background check (you may need to have your signature for this document witnessed by a notary public). You may even be asked if you have paid all state taxes!

You will need to note all your previous education/degrees. Some states might not be interested in your undergraduate education, but they will want to know your graduate education, including any post-master's credits/certificates. You will also need to supply official transcripts of all graduate education (usually in a sealed and signed envelope or emailed directly to the board). Although you will provide your graduate transcript(s), you will most likely need to complete an academic requirement form. The importance of making sure your graduate program matched the state's required course content was discussed earlier in this chapter. This is where you will need to "match" your courses with the state's course content areas, including demonstration of total credit hours. This form may also require the signature from your faculty advisor or program director. If you are applying from a well-known in-state program, then this form may be a formality (but still very important). If you are applying from out of state, the fit for each course with the appropriate content area may not always be clear. Thus, the board may ask you to provide a copy of your course syllabus. (Regardless of whether you are applying in state or out of state, it is always best to keep a copy of all your course syllabi. You never know if you will be asked to supply additional information about any courses taken.) With your educational experience, you will most likely need to provide the date you passed your licensing exam. Proof of evidence will need to be provided, often through an official score report.

Another important section of your application is documentation of your graduate counseling experience (i.e., practicum and internship) and your postgraduate counseling experience. As stated earlier, be sure you meet the minimum requirements (e.g., total number of hours, client hours, individual supervision hours, group supervision hours, client hours to supervision ratio). From the beginning of your training you should have also made sure that your supervisors meet the state's definition for an approved supervisor (if not, none of your hours will count!). Your supervisors will need to sign these documents as well. A helpful tip is to have your supervisors sign off on your hours soon after you complete your counseling experience. For example, have your practicum/internship supervisors sign off on your hours before you leave for a different agency for your job after graduation. It can sometimes be a significant challenge trying to obtain your past supervisors for their signatures (e.g., they no longer work at that agency, they moved out of state). If the state changes the counseling experience form from when you got your supervisor's signature to when you submit your application, you might need to get another signature with the new form.

In addition to your supervisors signing for your graduate and postgraduate counseling experience you may also need two or three professional references. These references often come from licensed mental health professionals, sometimes preferably from your postgraduate supervisor and any other most recent supervisor(s).

Finally, remember to sign the application and provide an application fee (often check or online credit card payment), which can range from $100 to $300. In most states, you will mail all the application materials together to the board's designated mailing address (some now have an online submission portal option). If you have appropriately submitted all your materials and the licensing board has no follow-up inquiries, you should hear back on their decision in one to three months. (The time frame for hearing back from the licensing board can vary greatly by state.) Once you hear back from the board and are informed that you are provisionally a licensed mental health counselor, you most likely will have to respond with another check (or online credit card payment) for your licensure fee. Do make sure you submit this licensure fee as soon as possible. You will most likely not be officially licensed until this fee is processed and you receive your license number (often printed on a card with your name). Finally, make sure to celebrate! Table 3.1 provides a summary of the key steps to obtain licensure, from graduate program requirements to the licensure application.

Table 3.1   Key Steps to Licensure

Criteria	Description
Graduate Program	Credit Hours • Most states require 48 or 60 • May need to receive all credits from the same program Course Content • Course name and content match state's required course content areas Accreditation • If required by state, is the program accredited (e.g., CACREP, MPCAC)? Practicum and Internship Training Opportunities • Practicum typically 100–200 hours • Internship typically 600–800 hours • Need to have approved licensed supervisor and meet required supervision hours and ratio of supervision hours to client hours Capstone Experience • Usually a thesis, comprehensive exam, or oral exam Consider: • Are students getting placements for their practicum/internships? • Are graduates getting jobs in reputable agencies after graduation? • Are graduates prepared/passing the licensure exam? • Are graduates getting licensed?

Postgraduate Experience	• Typically 2,000–4,000 hours, approximately two years full-time (three to four years part-time) • Need to have approved licensed supervisor and meet required supervision hours and ratio of supervision hours to client hours • Take note if state has multiple levels of licensure
Licensure Exam	• Determine if NCE, NCMHCE, and/or another licensure exam is required • Jurisprudence exam? • Alternative exam format (e.g., oral, essay, taped counseling session)? • Be sure to seek out study materials at NBCC's website and search the Internet; also consider state counseling association workshops and study groups
Application	• Personal information, including social security number, passport photo, past disciplinary action from licensing board, past felony or misdemeanor convictions, and criminal background check • Previous education/degrees, especially graduate education; including transcripts • Official score report indicating you passed your state's required licensing exam • Academic requirement form to match your graduate program courses with the state's required course content areas, including total credit hours • Documentation of your graduate counseling experience (i.e., practicum and internship) and your postgraduate counseling experience; be sure to meet the minimum requirements (e.g., total number of hours, direct hours, individual supervision hours, group supervision hours, client hours to supervision ratio) along with approved supervisors' signatures • Professional references usually from most recent supervisors • Sign and submit the application and provide the fee! • See Table 3.2 to avoid common application mistakes!

Common Licensure Application Mistakes

Some state licensing boards receive hundreds of applications a month, and it can take a few months to hear back on their decision for your application. Therefore, the last thing you want to do is make a mistake resulting in a "deficiency" requiring correction or additional information, or in the worst case, a rejection. According to the Massachusetts Mental Health Counseling Association (MaMHCA, 2019), the licensing board receives 85–100 license applications a month. Approximately 94% of those applications have some deficiency! Although many deficiencies can be relatively easily fixed, it can still be stressful and delay when you receive your license (possibly by many months). This slowdown could postpone a potential raise and/or delay/nullify a promotion or new employment opportunity. Table 3.2 provides a list of some of the more common mistakes one can make in one's licensure application. Some mistakes are simply a minor annoyance. Other mistakes can significantly delay receiving your license or possibly result in a denial.

Table 3.2   Common Licensure Application Mistakes

• Graduate program does not meet the state's required number of credit hours
• Did not obtain all required credits from the same graduate program (if required by state)
• Graduate courses do not meet the state's required course content
• Not including your graduate transcripts
• Client hours to supervision hours exceeds the required ratio (i.e., not enough supervision hours based on client hours)
• Supervisor does not qualify as an approved supervisor (i.e., not licensed, does not meet the board's definition of an approved supervisor, does not meet the post-licensure requirement)
• Not enough direct contact client hours (e.g., meet the total counseling hours criteria, but due to doing too many activities other than counseling)
• Not enough individual supervision hours (e.g., meet the total supervision hours criteria, but due to too many group supervision hours)
• Not meeting the required graduate counseling hours (i.e., practicum/internship)
• Submitting your application before obtaining the required total postgraduate counseling hours (or before minimum time frame)
• Documents without signature (e.g., application, criminal background check [or not witnessed/signed by a notary], counseling experience supervisor)
• Not providing your social security number (most states require this information for any type of licensure)
• Criminal background check is flagged for past offences, especially if not noted in your application up front
• Not including the application fee

Reflection Questions 3.4: Application for Licensure

- What are your thoughts and feelings about someday being in a position to submit your licensure application to the licensure board?
- What concerns do you have about completing any part of the licensure application?
- Are there any "common mistakes" that you think you may be prone to make? What can you do to avoid making those mistakes?

Activity 3.3: Preparing Licensure Application Materials

Obtain the application(s) for the state(s) you want to get licensed in. Use Appendix 1 for the state's website link and follow additional links, if necessary (most states provide their application as a pdf with instructions). Go through all the content to see how much matches up with what was just discussed in the previous section and what is different. Print out a copy of the application and start a "mock" application. Although at this point you are probably not ready to submit your application for review, you can complete many parts now (e.g., match the courses you have taken in your program with the state's course content areas, complete the practicum counseling experience document—and get it signed!). Keep this mock application on hand and complete more as you go. Because it is a mock application, you do not have to worry about making any mistakes. You can even take notes on the side for any reminders or thoughts for content that seems confusing. This process will help you figure out what still needs to be done and areas that might require some assistance. Overall, creating a mock application is an exposure process, which can demystify the experience, reduce anxiety, and help plan ahead to avoid any mistakes. Good luck!

LICENSE PORTABILITY

Some organizations have been working together (i.e., American Association of State Counseling Boards [AASCB], AMHCA, Association for Counselor Education and Supervision [ACES], CACREP, and NBCC) on expanding the potential option of license portability (sometimes called reciprocity) between states (see AMHCA, 2021). Portability means that your license in one state would be accepted to receive licensure in another state. In other words, perhaps you are licensed (e.g., LMHC or LPC) in one state and you move to another state. You would still have to complete some form of licensure application, but you would not have to worry about particular nuances (e.g., an additional course, a few extra practicum hours, a different licensure exam) if the licensure board has determined that the licensure requirements are effectively the same between the two states. Essentially, your license would naturally transfer from one state to another. This situation would make your life a lot easier when moving from one state to another. However, each state varies greatly in its education and training requirements (or limits) on portability. Thus, it would be prudent to contact the licensing board of the state you plan on moving to in advance to know the specific requirements. Some states are explicit in identifying specific states they have portability agreements with. Other states will simply say that they review applications on a case-by-case basis. This means you might not know if you are able to immediately get licensed, or have to meet additional requirements, until after you submit your application and hear back from the licensing board.

Chapter 4 addresses the topic of professional advocacy. This is a great example of an issue to advocate for the counseling profession. Not only can portability benefit yourself and your colleagues by allowing for an easier process to get licensed in other states, it can also benefit the public. For example, there are millions of Americans who live in locations across the US (especially rural areas) where there is a shortage of qualified mental health counselors (AMHCA, 2021). There are also populations that belong to particular minority groups, those experiencing poverty, and senior citizens where access to quality mental health care is limited (AMHCA, 2021). There are many licensed mental health counselors who would consider moving to another state to help serve such populations but are hesitant because they think (or know for a fact) that their license will not easily transfer over. Allowing for portability will allow greater professional flexibility for many mental health counselors. Such flexibility can expand the reach of the counseling profession, especially to those most in need.

REFERENCES

Alliance for Professional Counselors. (2021). Mission and Goals. Retrieved January 25, 2021, from https://apccounseloralliance.org/about-us/mission-and-goals/

American Mental Health Counselors Association. (2021). National Counselor Licensure Endorsement Process. Retrieved January 27, 2021, from http://www.amhca.org/advocacy/portability

Buckman, L. R., Nordal, K. C., & DeMers, S. T. (2018). Regulatory and licensure issues derived from the summit on master's training in psychological practice. *Professional Psychology: Research and Practice, 49*, 321–326. https://doi.org/10.1037/pro0000214

Campbell, L. F., Worrell, F. C., Dailey, A. T., & Brown, R. T. (2018). Master's level practice: Introduction, history, and current status. *Professional Psychology: Research and Practice, 49*, 299–305. http://dx.doi.org/10.1037/pro0000202

Hughes, T. L., & Diaz-Granados, J. (2018). Master's summit: Quality assurance and accreditation. *Professional Psychology: Research and Practice, 49*, 306–310. https://doi.org/10.1037/pro0000199

Massachusetts Mental Health Counseling Association (MaMHCA). (2019). MaMHCA helping with back-log at licensing board. *MaMHCA Newsletter, 38*(4).

Masters in Psychology and Counseling Accreditation Council. (2021). Frequently Asked Questions. Retrieved January 25, 2021, from http://mpcacaccreditation.org/faq/

National Board of Certified Counselors. (2021). Examinations. Retrieved January 27, 2021, from https://www.nbcc.org/Exams

ADDITIONAL RESOURCES

Academy of Cognitive and Behavioral Therapies website: www.academyofct.org

Beck Institute website: www.beckinstitute.org

CPH & Associates webpage for counselors: https://www.cphins.com/counselor/

Healthcare Providers Service Organization webpage for counselors: http://www.hpso.com/individuals/professional-liability/malpractice-insurance-for-counselors

Mometrix Test Prep. (2016). *NCE secrets study guide: NCE exam review for the National Counselor Examination*. Author.

Mometrix Test Prep. (2020). *NCMHCE secrets study guide: Exam review and NCMHCE practice test for the National Clinical Mental Health Counseling Examination* (2nd ed.). Author.

TPB Publishing. (2020). *NCE exam preparation study guide: NCE exam prep and practice test questions* (3rd ed.). Author.

TPB Publishing. (2020). *NCMHCE study guide: NCMHCE exam prep and practice test questions for the National Clinical Mental Health Counseling Examination* (2nd ed.). Author.

4

Expectations beyond Counseling

■ ■ ■

Obviously, part of being a good mental health counselor is having excellent therapeutic skills. However, being a successful counselor goes well beyond what happens in the counseling room with your clients. There are many logistical components to consider, from completing paperwork to working with a variety of other professionals, some of whom may not be counselors. In other words, you will need to have good interpersonal and documentation skills. (Yes, that means good communication and writing skills.) There may eventually come a time when you will be a supervisor or administrator, which requires advanced clinical and organizational skills. Simply put, there is a lot more to being a mental health counselor than counseling.

As will be discussed in Chapter 6, much of the stress of being a mental health counselor does not come directly from your clients; it comes from the nature of the field. The reality is that you will most likely be dedicating as much time to bureaucratic responsibilities (or annoyances) as to your counseling responsibilities. Much of the stress comes from the time pressure associated with caring for your clients while also trying to maneuver your way through agency politics, difficult colleagues, outside providers, and nonstop paperwork. The expectations beyond counseling addressed in this chapter include paperwork, case management, colleagues, supervision, managed care organizations, mental health community outreach, and professional advocacy. This information is not meant to scare you, but rather to provide a clear and honest picture of the many responsibilities of a mental health counselor. My hope is that, instead of feeling shocked and ambushed, you will be prepared (as much as you can be) for the full expectations well beyond what goes on in the counseling room.

PAPERWORK

All mental health settings require documentation of many tasks. This results in a lot of paperwork. This paperwork is unavoidable. (The word paperwork will be used to encompass all forms of documentation, knowing that much of it is now completed electronically—i.e., electronic work.) Some of the most common types of paperwork for mental health counselors include intake assessments, case formulations and treatment plans, progress notes, and discharge summaries. Please note that the focus here is not on how to complete each of these forms (that is best suited for a text on counseling skills). Rather, the emphasis is on highlighting the common content of these forms of documentation and their central role in providing the best care possible for your clients. Appropriate documentation through paperwork is a must. Not completing your paperwork (and not on time) is poor care at best and unethical at worst.

It should be noted here that you will eventually have to become acquainted with the Health Insurance Portability and Accountability Act (HIPAA). HIPAA is a federal law enacted by Congress in 1996 to protect personal health information, including appropriate security measures, and provides rights concerning the release of such information (U.S. Department of Health and Human Services, 2021). Although HIPAA is well beyond the scope of this text, it is important to note that it covers all documentation requirements that must be followed for insurance and confidentiality purposes. Of course, in addition to HIPAA rule, you will have to know the documentation requirements of each managed care organization (MCO) for your clients and any legal statutes specific to the state you are providing services in. Any agency you would be employed by will need to follow HIPAA.

Intake Assessment

Before clients have their first session, they typically need to complete some paperwork on their own, including informed consent documents and confidentiality waivers. Soon afterward, you are able to meet with them for 50–60 minutes to complete an intake assessment during your first session (you may need another session to complete). The specific name and content for this process can vary greatly by agency. Nevertheless, your goal is to collect historical information (e.g., family history, past significant events, prior treatment), indicators of current functioning (e.g., reported symptoms, daily activities, quality of relationships with others), and their perspective of what they want to get out of counseling. You may also use additional formal assessments that provide global indicators of distress or specific syndromes of distress. The goal of this intake assessment process is to gather as much relevant information as possible related to your clients' presenting distress.

An intake assessment is a time when note taking is a must while you are asking a multitude of semi-structured questions. Your agency will have specific questions you must answer, but you will also most likely have some leeway to ask follow-up questions specific to your clients' presenting distress as you gather more information. Often, the information garnered from the intake assessment will be needed to develop a formal diagnosis, which is required by MCOs to continue providing services. This means you will typically have no more than one week to complete the intake assessment. Furthermore, your intake assessment will also greatly inform your eventual case formulation and treatment plan. Thus, your goal here is to be as efficient and detailed as possible.

Case Formulation and Treatment Plan

Even while doing your intake assessment, it is essential that you also conceptualize how your clients developed their current distress. Within about 2–3 weeks of completing your intake assessment, you will need to complete a case formulation and treatment plan for your clients. It is best to get this done sooner than later, as this will be the driving force behind what you do in session. It will give you purpose and structure to your counseling sessions; a must for effectively improving client well-being. A case formulation (sometimes called a case conceptualization) is a client narrative that integrates historical information and current functioning to provide an explanation of current mental health distress and presenting problems. Its primary goal is to provide a hypothesis of contributing factors to their current ways of thinking, feeling, and behaving. Most of the time, this information is synthesized through a theoretical lens and matches the client's presenting problems and diagnosis. Again, the style, theoretical lens, and the aspects of the client's life that are emphasized will vary by agency. Although a case formulation can be modified as counseling progresses, it is important to provide a substantively detailed case formulation early in counseling. What you write will not only influence your treatment plan, it will also influence how you perceive your clients and proceed early in counseling.

Your treatment plan will need to match your case formulation. In other words, there should be goals and interventions that address the contributing factors and effects of the client's presenting problems. Treatment plans can also identify potential obstacles to counseling, client's strengths, and recommendations for additional services (e.g., psychological assessment, group counseling, medication referral). Of course, your treatment plan should have the same theoretical lens as your case formulation. Ideally, a good treatment plan provides a blueprint of how counseling will proceed by way of interventions, including clear indicators of progress. This means your treatment goals should be measurable, specific, attainable, and time-limited. This helps not only you and your client track treatment progress, but also MCOs. As a caveat, it is best to make sure that your interventions are evidence-based in relation to the client's presenting problems and diagnosis. Ideally, you should also receive feedback from your clients on the case formulation and collaboratively develop their treatment plan. The more your clients are on board with your treatment approach, the better the chance to establish a strong therapeutic alliance and enhance treatment progress. Overall, it can take considerable thought and time to develop a solid case formulation and treatment plan, especially for early-career counselors. With that said, your case formulation and treatment plan are not "set in stone." Revisions can be made over time to either document as you obtain additional information and treatment progresses. In fact, many agencies require quarterly (sometimes monthly) case formulation and treatment plan reviews. In the end, developing a case formulation and treatment plan is a vital skill for mental health counselors. This skill positively correlates with providing effective counseling.

Progress Note

Every time you have a counseling session with a client, you will be required to provide written documentation of the treatment provided. The exact content of a progress note varies greatly based on agency and MCOs. At the very least, you will be required to document the nature of the contact, type of service provided, disposition of the client (behavioral indicators are best), key topics discussed (at least generally), and treatment goals focused on with associated interventions. Some agencies require a more standardized format, such as SOAP (Subjective, Objective, Assessment, and Plan). Overall, there should be enough information in the progress note to remind you of key indicators to inform your next session. Other contacts with your client and service providers (e.g., phone calls, assessment reviews, treatment plan reviews, consultations) are sometimes also included as a progress note (sometimes referred to as a case management note).

A single progress note for each session may not sound like a challenging task; by itself this is usually true. However, when seeing thirty or more clients each week, many times back-to-back, along with attending to many other obligations, this can be very challenging. It is important to complete these progress notes as soon as possible. More times than not, these progress notes are necessary to document services rendered to get reimbursed through MCOs. Furthermore, the contents of the progress notes are important to inform yourself on how to proceed for the next session and future treatment planning. These progress notes allow you to track the "progress" your clients are making toward improved mental health.

Some agencies require concurrent progress notes. What this means is that you complete the progress note while in session with your client. This process may even involve live input from your client. In some ways, this is an efficient way to complete a progress note; your paperwork is completed when the session is done. However, some counselors may find that this is distracting for implementing interventions and possibly interferes with the counselor–client relationship. Another option is to complete the progress note immediately after the session is complete. Technically, if you have an hour-long session with a client, it is really supposed to be approximately 45–50 minutes (again, the exact time varies by agencies and MCOs), with the remaining time used for progress notes. Some counselors can do this rather well, while others struggle because it requires beginning and ending each session on time and self-discipline to compete the progress note. This can be easier said than done when seeing multiple back-to-back clients, especially if an earlier session starts or ends late (i.e., it can have a cascading effect). What some counselors end up doing is trying to complete all their progress notes at the end of the day or the following morning. Unfortunately, this is not ideal because after a long day of 6–8+ clients, remembering key details can be difficult, especially if the note is completed on the following day. The general rule is to go no more than 24 hours after a session to complete a progress note. Some supervisors and agencies may consider anything over 24–48 hours as unethical. Unfortunately, it is not that uncommon to hear counselors report that they are a week or more behind on their progress notes. This is very concerning because, as stated earlier, the information in each progress note is important to make future treatment decisions. Over time this can result in providing counseling sessions with little to no direction and purpose, resulting in very poor client care. Ultimately, you will have to discover the best way to complete your progress notes based on your agency's expectations and your own style. Whatever your approach, it is best to have a reliable system in place that allows for progress note completion as soon as possible.

Discharge Plan and Summary

There will eventually come a time when you will need to discontinue services with your clients. Ideally, most of the time it will be because counseling was successful and your clients are ready to "terminate" and move forward on their own (i.e., treatment goals were/will be obtained). Other times counseling may be terminated because a predetermined number of sessions has been reached as specified by the clients' MCO, clients no longer want services or are no longer benefitting, or a referral to another provider (e.g., someone better trained to meet the clients' needs) and/or continuing care (e.g., a different level of treatment like a hospital inpatient setting) is necessary.

Regardless of the reason for termination, it is important to be continually assessing your clients' progress throughout treatment so you can adjust your counseling interventions and therapeutic relationship. Many agencies now require a discharge plan and summary to make this process more purposeful and clear to the clients. Sometimes you have many weeks (or months) to plan ahead; other times the termination may be abrupt (within a few days). There is less consistency across agencies in what is required in a discharge plan and summary. Some of the more common elements include remaining goals/interventions before termination, description of overall treatment progress since counseling started, formal statement of reason to terminate, recommendations, possible future problems (or prognosis), level of functioning at termination, and possible referrals. This information is important to document because it will be helpful for any referrals to maintain a proper level of continuing care. It is also possible that clients will require counseling in the future, either at your agency, or another agency. Thus, it is important that clients' future providers are aware of prior counseling, including their status at termination.

Reflection Questions 4.1: Paperwork Challenges

- What are your thoughts about having to complete extensive paperwork for each client?
- Why is it important to keep all paperwork up-to-date for each client?
- What are some possible challenges (personal or agency related) to completing paperwork on time?
- What are some ways to plan/organize your work day to ensure a good-faith effort to complete paperwork on time?

CASE MANAGEMENT

Outside of counseling and doing paperwork, there are often a lot of behind-the-scenes activities that you will do for some of your clients. What you do, and how much you do, will vary greatly by agency and population served. Some clients you will see once a week for counseling, completing the appropriate paperwork afterwards. For others, you might spend more time on the phone and in meetings with other providers. A formal definition of case management is the overall maintenance of your clients' psychological, physical, and social environment with the goals of facilitating reduced mental health distress, personal growth, physical survival, and possible community involvement. A more informal definition of case management is "all that other stuff" you do besides counseling. (Technically some may consider paperwork as part of case management as well, but the focus here is beyond direct counseling-related activities.) In addition to supplemental mental health referrals, case management includes assistance with medical care, employment/unemployment services, school/education services, disability services, social services, food pantries, domestic violence shelters, housing, transportation, family/social relationships, social justice advocacy, legal system, and other community participation (and much more!). Essentially, good case management is an ongoing process that consists of assessing clients' needs and coordinating with other providers and community-based services to supplement and enhance quality of care.

Many early-career mental health counselors are surprised to learn of all the duties associated with case management, as their expectations are to do primarily counseling; even some level of paperwork is expected. Some may even complain that they feel like a social worker. However, it is important to realize that some clients need more help beyond counseling. A competent mental health counselor truly follows a holistic approach. This does not mean you will be doing all of these tasks on your own, but you can at least put them in the right direction with the appropriate resources and continuous monitoring.

It might be helpful to look at it this way: only so much change can realistically happen in counseling. Many times, particular types of clients' change require assistance from other professionals, particular aspects of the system, and their surrounding environment. Furthermore, consider Maslow's hierarchy of needs. It is hard to talk about esteem needs when physiological needs are a concern. In other words, basic needs must be met first, and maintained, in order to accomplish some of your counseling goals. For example, it is not realistic to expect clients to focus on identifying negative automatic thoughts if they have genuine concerns about where they are going to sleep that night. Your role in your clients' lives is especially unique. In many cases, you are a vital link between your clients and the care delivery system.

Reflection Questions 4.2: Case Management Expectations

- What are your thoughts about having to go beyond counseling for some of your clients?
- What do you think would be the most challenging aspect of case management for you?
- How could not meeting your clients' basic needs impact the effectiveness of counseling?

WORKING WITH COLLEAGUES

The stress of being a mental health counselor due to the nature of the field and agencies is addressed in Chapter 6. One aspect that can be both rewarding and frustrating is working with colleagues who have many different roles in the care of your clients. In many ways it is great to work with other professionals, both within and outside the counseling field, who also have a vested interest in your clients. A lot can be learned from understanding different perspectives of presenting problems and approaches to care. In fact, some of the ideas and thoughts from these professionals can have a positive influence on your future counseling sessions. Other times, it can be challenging when multiple providers have varying perspectives that may appear to be in conflict with each other. This can also include working with providers who may have difficult personalities and communication styles.

Inside your agency, you will be working with colleagues on site (i.e., coworkers) on a nearly day-to-day basis. Depending on your agency, this can include other counselors (with a variety of different training backgrounds and degrees), psychologists, psychiatrists, nurses, residential staff, and educators. Often, meetings within your agency are for treatment teams, case consultations, in-service trainings, or supervision (individual or group). Outside your agency (i.e., outside providers), you may find yourself working with social workers, education administrators, state mental/public health workers, physicians, law enforcement, probation officers, attorneys, and any of the individuals noted working within your agency. Most of the time, when you work with professionals outside your agency it is for continuing care consultation or for a formal meeting to discuss matters that may have a different focus than primarily counseling (e.g., education needs, medical concerns, legal status, custody). Ideally, all providers should be working collaboratively for the best care possible for their clients. Unfortunately, working with multiple different providers can sometimes result in approaches (and agendas) that you do not believe are in the best interest of your clients. You may also be the only mental health expert in these meetings. In such cases, it is important to know your role while respectfully advocating for the best interests of your clients.

Regardless of what you think of your coworkers or outside providers, you will have to learn to get along with them as best you can. Similar to your family, you are often unable to choose your colleagues. This does not mean you must be "best friends" with every colleague, but it does mean you should conduct yourself in a professional manner. Sometimes we spend more time with our colleagues than with family or friends. Thus, it makes sense to have at least a decent relationship. This approach will make your role as a counselor, and life in general, more pleasant. If it helps, consider how your own well-being and professional demeanor are important for maintaining the best interests of your clients.

As silly as it may sound, consider using many of your client counselor skills with your colleagues, if necessary. Remember, being a good mental health counselor goes well beyond your counseling and paperwork skills. Just as you do with your clients, try to build rapport with your colleagues, especially those you work closest with. Be respectful to others, even if you are not treated respectfully yourself; do your best to take the high road. Avoid offensive/sarcastic talk and behaviors, including spreading rumors. Do your best to be sincerely friendly on a daily basis, including socializing, smiling, and small acts of kindness. Also, be open to feedback and advice. This does not mean you have to agree; just listen and do not be defensive. Finally, it really helps your image if you come off not only as friendly but also as a conscientious and reliable colleague. Nothing helps your work relationships more than being a competent, pleasant, and dependable colleague.

Reflection Questions 4.3: Working with Colleagues Challenges

- What are your initial thoughts about working with a variety of colleagues from different training backgrounds and perspectives on client care?
- What type of colleague personality trait or behavior would be the most difficult for you to work with? Would could you do about it?
- What are your best personal traits that you could build on to establish and enhance good working relationships with your colleagues?
- What personal traits would you need to monitor and possibly improve upon to work effectively with your colleagues?

SUPERVISION

You should expect to be supervised at any agency where you provide counseling, especially while in training (i.e., practicum and internship) and postgraduate while working toward licensure. Ideally, even after you are licensed it is important to continue receiving supervision. Typically, you will be supervised by at least one colleague who has more years of experience than you and is licensed. However, in some agencies you may also have a secondary supervisor. Furthermore, you will most likely receive group supervision, which may involve the same supervisor you see individually or someone different. Supervision is addressed in more detail in Chapter 3 within the context of licensure and in Chapter 7 as part of your professional development. The focus here is to provide a basic, general explanation of what to expect.

You will typically formally meet with your supervisor for supervision at least 1–2 hours a week. Group supervision is also at least 1–2 hours a week, and a secondary supervisor is about 1 hour a week. While in training and postgraduate pre-licensure, you are working under your supervisor's license. This means that your supervisor is acting as a gatekeeper to the profession while constantly monitoring the quality of professional services you offer to your clients (along with your documentation skills and overall general conduct with other colleagues). As a gatekeeper, your supervisor will ultimately be making evaluative decisions that can impact your future training and graduation. This is a hierarchical relationship that is in place not only for your professional development but also to ensure that the well-being of clients is protected.

In most cases (ideally all), supervisors do their best to nurture your development and want to see you succeed and move up through the profession. Your supervisor will spend much time acquainting you to the profession, including some of the topics discussed in this chapter (e.g., paperwork, case management, MCOs). They will also assist you with understanding the basic day-to-day activities (e.g., treatment team meetings, intake assessments). Of course, there will be a heavy focus on your work with clients, ranging from basic counseling skills to skills specific to your theoretical orientation. Preferably, part of your supervision should include reviewing audio/video of your counseling sessions. Sometimes supervision can also incorporate live observation and feedback. You can also verbally report your counseling with clients, but this is not the optimal scenario for accurate self-reporting and effective counseling skill development (Bartle-Haring et al., 2009; Champe & Kleist, 2003). Sometimes, supervisors will demonstrate particular counselor skills by having you observe their sessions (live or recorded) or through role-plays (group supervision works well for this). Your supervisor is also typically the first one you report to for an agency concern or a client crisis (e.g., suicidal ideation). Finally, there should also be a focus on having a strong understanding of professional ethics, multicultural awareness, and some personal introspection. Although the supervision process may sound intimidating, it is a great opportunity for you to grow as a mental health counselor and as an individual. Finally, pay attention to the strengths and limitations of your supervisors. You may someday be a supervisor yourself soon after receiving your license. Your experiences as a supervisee along with additional training will go a long way in shaping your supervision skills. Do not assume being a "good counselor" naturally translates into being a "good supervisor."

Reflection Questions 4.4: Supervision Thoughts

- Do you feel intimidated/threatened/insecure about the thought of being supervised? Explain your thoughts and feelings.
- What do you think you could gain most about being a mental health counselor from supervision?
- What personal and professional supervisor qualities are the most important to you?
- Knowing your personality and work ethic, how do you think you will respond to supervision?

MANAGED CARE ORGANIZATIONS

Almost any agency you work for will have a working relationship with Managed Care Organizations (MCOs). How much direct contact you have with MCOs as an early-career clinical mental counselor will vary by agency. Regardless, it is helpful to have at least a basic understanding of MCOs when you begin seeing clients, especially because there has been a major expansion of MCOs over the past 10–15 years. Few things in the mental health field have had as significant an impact on access and providing counseling services as the managed care movement. MCOs will most likely continue to be the norm for many years ahead.

In short, MCOs provide third-party reimbursement for mental health and physical health services. Typically, large health care corporations are in a position to determine the cost (i.e., financing) and delivery of health services. Most people sign up for a specific type of health care plan provided by their employer. The overarching goal of MCOs is to reduce costs while increasing the quality of care (i.e., management). (This was largely in response to the exorbitant fee-for-service systems in place prior to the 1980s.) A common word used by MCOs is "efficiency." However, not all health care plans are equal in available care and costs. Thus, working with each MCO will have its own idiosyncrasies.

In order to get reimbursed for counseling sessions from MCOs you will first need to obtain what is called "authorization." Most MCOs require that you obtain pre-authorization before any services can be provided. A pre-authorization typically requires an Outpatient Treatment Report (OTR), which includes providing key information about the client's presentation and need for treatment. The OTR is looked at as an initial treatment plan (although your agency may have its own formal treatment plan). You will get the information for the OTR from your intake assessment. In most cases, you will need to provide a formal diagnosis before you can have your first counseling session after the intake assessment. The OTR will also be used in the future to request additional counseling sessions.

For MCOs you will need to make sure that your treatment goals are measurable, specific, attainable, time-limited, and are appropriately matched by your interventions. This includes some level of indication of how your client will be different and improved at the conclusion of treatment. Furthermore, as discussed earlier, you will need to keep a record of each of your counseling sessions, known as progress notes. You need to have documentation, or "proof," that a session was conducted and that it matches your treatment goals and interventions to get reimbursed (Sutton, 2015). Overall, brief counseling approaches are often preferred because MCOs focus on both cost and time efficiency (Eaves et al., 2008; Lawless et al., 1999; Talbott, 2001).

While providing counseling, MCOs engage in ongoing monitoring, which can require additional documentation of treatment. A more formal term for this process is utilization review (UR). More specifically, UR follows stipulated standards to assess treatment needs (including diagnosis), appropriateness of treatment goals and interventions, and overall treatment effectiveness. UR technically initiates before counseling begins (i.e., intake assessment and OTR; "potential"), during counseling ("simultaneous"), and after counseling ends ("retrospective"). In some instances, you may be required to interact directly with an MCO UR representative to provide a rationale for the treatment provided, which may also include a request for additional sessions. Sometimes the UR representative may offer treatment suggestions or not authorize additional sessions. This can be understandably frustrating, considering the UR representative does not know the full contextual picture of your client and may not even be trained and/or experienced in providing counseling.

Ultimately, many mental health counselors report dissatisfaction working with MCOs, including compromising their standards of practice and being in contradiction to compliance with their professional code of ethics (Cohen et al., 2006; Danzinger & Welfel, 2001; Rosenberg & DeMaso, 2008). The focus of this chapter is not to get into the politics of working with MCOs. However, it is important to highlight some of the more common frustrations working with MCOs to provide a clearer contextual understanding of the process. Broadly, because of the UR process, some counselors feel restricted in their ability to care for their clients because they do not have full freedom to implement their treatment approaches as desired. This can put counselors in a difficult position because they may either need to follow the UR representative suggestions (which may be believed to be inappropriate or unethical) or possibly risk not being reimbursed and/or not authorized for future sessions. This puts counselors in a position to balance their relationship with MCOs with the welfare of their clients, including any potential ethical dilemmas. Ultimately, mental health counselors should be advocates for their clients and do their best to present a sound argument for additional counseling sessions and/or continuing to follow established treatment goals.

Related to treatment plans, there have also been concerns about the overemphasis on the medical model of necessity, especially with regard to focusing on diagnoses, which can further pathologize clients (Cooper & Gottlieb, 2000). In part, this is the reason why MCOs sometimes dictate particular treatment approaches for specific diagnostic categories. The focus is less on life enhancement and overall well-being, and more on finding a diagnosis for the "problem(s)." As stated earlier, MCOs will not authorize sessions for reimbursement if an eligible diagnosis is not provided. Furthermore, the number of authorized sessions will vary by both MCO and diagnosis. This can result in limiting options for individualized client care. Unfortunately, this can result in counselors being put in a bind between reporting an accurate diagnosis that may result in not being reimbursed and an inaccurate diagnosis to get reimbursed. As unprofessional as changing a diagnosis may sound, it does occur within the counseling profession. For example, Danzinger and Welfel's (2001) survey of licensed mental health counselors found that 44% had changed or would consider changing a diagnosis to obtain MCO reimbursement. Of course, deliberate misdiagnosing for any reason violates ACA's and AMHCA's code of ethics. Furthermore, it is also illegal as it constitutes insurance fraud.

There are also concerns about MCOs negatively affecting the counselor–client therapeutic relationship, including confidentiality (Cooper & Gottlieb, 2000). Typically, clients should feel comfortable sharing any of their thoughts or feelings without being concerned that their information could go beyond the counseling room (unless the client is a risk to harm self or others, of course). However, sometimes particularly sensitive client information may need to be shared with MCOs for treatment necessity as part of the UR. Additionally, once this information is shared with MCOs, it is no longer under your control. Of course, ethically, clients should be made aware of how their MCO will be involved in their treatment and their right/privilege to release confidential information (i.e., HIPAA). This can potentially inhibit what clients share, affecting not only the therapeutic relationship but also treatment effectiveness (Cohen et al., 2006; Danzinger & Welfel, 2001).

Overall, it is important to keep in mind that providing counseling to clients and working with MCOs is a business. MCOs are in a position to be efficient, by way of reducing cost and increasing quality of care.

Unfortunately, this approach to efficiency can sometimes result in disagreements between mental health counselors and MCOs about client quality of care. In some cases, these differences can result in loss of autonomy and potential ethical dilemmas. Thus, it is important for counselors to be strong advocates for their clients while still upholding their professional ethical standards (see Wolff & Schlesinger, 2002; Rosenberg & DeMaso, 2008).

Reflection Questions 4.5: Managed Care Organizations Concerns

- What are your thoughts on MCOs' role in efficiency (i.e., reducing cost while increasing quality of care)?
- What are your thoughts on balancing your relationship with MCOs and advocating for your clients, especially about appropriate treatment goals/interventions and requesting additional sessions?
- It is unethical to change a client's diagnosis for reimbursement of services. What would be the motivation for some counselors to consider this option? What are some alternative, ethical options to consider?
- What are your concerns about client confidentiality when working with MCOs? How can client concerns about MCO confidentiality affect the therapeutic relationship and treatment effectiveness?

MENTAL HEALTH COMMUNITY OUTREACH

Community outreach can be a very broad topic and has received increasing attention as a primary focus of treatment over the past decade (see Burns & Firn, 2017; Williams et al., 2011); it is sometimes now referred to as "assertive community outreach." Here, the focus is on emphasizing the importance and possible expectation by agencies to connect locally with their community in order to provide services of most need. A key reason to engage in mental health community outreach is to help destigmatize the topic and provide resources to help reduce their distress. Although mental health issues are gaining more attention, their overall recognition is still relatively minimal compared to medical conditions. No matter what community you work in, at least some (or many) will have mental health needs. It only makes sense for agencies to be aware of the mental health needs that affect the communities they practice in.

Many agencies now expect their mental health counselors to engage in activities that reduce the stigma of mental health while also offering services and/or providing referrals. Of course, what services you provide can greatly vary depending on the community your agency serves and the expertise of the counselors. Examples of common disorders/problem areas for outreach include major depressive disorder, bipolar disorder, generalized anxiety disorder, posttraumatic stress disorder, obsessive-compulsive disorders, eating disorders, body image, substance abuse, self-harm, neurodevelopmental disorders, social skills, and bullying. Examples of common populations include children/adolescents, peri/postnatal mental health, LGBTQ+, elderly, racial/ethnic minorities, immigrants, veterans, and disabled. Examples of common settings include community centers, recreation centers, schools (pre-K to secondary), colleges/universities, businesses, nursing homes, and elderly care facilities.

The only way to truly know your community's needs will be to do some form of assessment. This may include an agency having counselors ask individuals in the community to complete surveys (local mailing list, including organizations) or to actually go out into the community and talk to different leaders (high school principal, CEO of LGBTQ+ center, director of nursing home). It is important to know this information going into an agency that does mental health community outreach so that you are aware you may be communicating with other people besides other counselors and professionals outside of mental health. Consider approaching directors of a nursing home to help them understand the relevance of possible presenting concerns (e.g., forms of dementia, loneliness, anxiety) while also demonstrating and motivating them to recognize your agency as a possible source to address this need. In other words, although you can certainly use some of your counseling communication skills, you will also have to adapt how you explain particular presenting concerns (i.e., reduced jargon, relatable) while also demonstrating competence.

Another way agencies may engage with the community is to host/participate in a local event with other mental health professionals that includes speakers on topics of interest while also providing resources and referrals. For example, May is Mental Health Awareness Month, which could be a good time to host a series of mental health topics at the local community center. Of course, many agencies participate in community engagement throughout the year. Relatedly, there may be other larger/broader community events where your agency can rent a booth or space to promote your agency while also providing brief psychoeducation about mental health topics to those who are interested.

The National Institute of Mental Health (NIMH, 2021) has an extensive Outreach Partnership Program. It is a nationwide initiative to increase public awareness of evidence-based mental health information. A select group of community mental health organizations serve as NIMH Outreach Partners with the goal of educating the public about mental health and related research. The NIMH Outreach Partnership Program web page has additional links for excellent resources related to community outreach and related research.

Activity 4.1: Mental Health Outreach in Your Community

Get into a small group of peers and discuss the potential mental health needs of the communities that you live in (or where you are completing your practicum/internship, if applicable). Consider making a list of disorders/problems, populations, and settings that are in need of mental health support. Consider the following:

- What is the evidence, or rationale, for your noted disorders/problems, populations, and settings within your community? In other words, how do you know (or at least think) these are the needs of your community that deserve the most attention?
- What are some feasible options for community outreach for your above-noted needs?
- What would be some potential obstacles in implementing your community outreach?
- What are your thoughts about being asked by your agency to engage in mental health community outreach? Is this something that aligns with your approach to mental health counseling? Do you have any concerns?

PROFESSIONAL ADVOCACY

It has been stated a few times in this chapter about your role as an advocate for your clients. You will eventually find yourself in a position to advocate for the counseling profession as well as for your clients. Advocacy in this context refers to taking action and supporting particular policies and standards for the profession. Obviously, professional advocacy can also promote client/social advocacy beyond the counseling room; they complement each other. Essentially, if the profession of counseling is respected and recognized as credible by the public and other related professions, then mental health counselors can become strong advocates. Also important is how the counseling profession is perceived by legislators, MCOs, and employers, which can result in more effective lobbying efforts and greater resources to support the mental and social health of your clients. In sum, being an advocate for systemic change in both the counseling profession and society at large can benefit the well-being of your clients.

As an early-career counselor, it may be initially challenging to get involved in advocacy tasks due to your lack of experience. As you gain more counseling and systemic experience, you will develop a more robust professional identity and eventually find particular deficiencies of concern, typically at the community or state level. Such experiences will make you a more informed advocate with an expanded social network to get your voice heard. If you ever find yourself feeling despondent when you notice a systemic flaw compromising the integrity of the counseling profession and/or client well-being, do your best to avoid cynicism. Your "single voice" may become a "loud yell" as you discover that many other counseling professionals have the same concerns.

It is highly recommended that you join your state's mental health counseling association. The state level is where you may have the strongest impact and most immediate results. Much change can be made at the state level, and over time, it can have an influence at the national level as other states follow suit (similar to other types of social change). One current example in Massachusetts at the time of publication of this book is "HB 1705: An Act of Expanding Access and Safety of Mental Health Services" (Massachusetts Mental Health Counselors Association, 2021). The goal of this legislation is to allow hospitalization privileges (i.e., "Section 12 Privileges Parity Bill") for licensed mental health counselors. Currently in Massachusetts, physicians, psychologists, psychiatrist nurse mental health clinical specialists, licensed independent clinical social workers, and police officers have hospitalization privileges. The argument is that licensed mental health counselors have equivalent (or greater) education and training relative to that of current covered providers. This also provides the best care possible for clients, as it allows for their needs to be immediately met rather than waiting for another co-professional to "sign off."

At the national level, the American Counseling Association (ACA) and the American Mental Health Counseling Association (AMHCA) are two of the most active and well-known organizations that advocate for mental health counselors. There are times when advocacy at the national level can have a significant impact on the profession in your home state (e.g., The Mental Health Parity and Addiction Equity Act of 2008). One current example at the time of publication of this book is licensure portability (also discussed in Chapter 3). Simply stated, portability allows a licensed mental health counselor in one state to be recognized to practice in another state. Currently, it can sometimes be challenging to maintain licensure when a mental health counselor moves from one state to another, due to variations in state education and training requirements. In addition to creating consistent licensure standards across states, this proposal establishes minimum standards for safe practice and can increase public access to high-quality care (AMHCA, 2021a). One final example is the AMHCA (2021b) sponsored Capitol Hill Briefing entitled "Access to Mental Health Care in Rural

America: A Crisis in the Making for Seniors and People with Disabilities." Currently, psychiatrists, psychologists, mental health clinical nurse specialists, and clinical social workers are listed as Medicare-covered providers. However, mental health counselors are not included, even though the profession has equivalent (or greater) education and training relative to that of current covered providers. Overall, these few state and national examples of legislation advocacy highlight the importance of establishing the credibility of the counseling profession, which in turn results in high-quality care for our clients. For additional information on professional advocacy, the ACA (2021) website provides some good resources (e.g., election tool kit, advocacy tips, effective meetings, social media).

Reflection Questions 4.6: Social Advocacy Involvement

- What are your thoughts about getting involved in politics/legislation at the community, state, or national level?
- Based upon your own skills, what way do you think you could be most helpful in advocating for the mental health counseling profession?
- As an early-career mental health counselor, have you already noticed any systemic concerns at the community, state, or national level that may require advocacy?

REFERENCES

American Counseling Association. (2021). Government Affairs: Advocacy Tips and Tools. Retrieved January 21, 2021, from https://www.counseling.org/government-affairs/advocacy-tips-tools

American Mental Health Counselors Association. (2021a). National Counselor Licensure Endorsement Process. Retrieved January 21, 2021, from http://www.amhca.org/advocacy/portability

American Mental Health Counselors Association. (2021b). Take Action on HR.945 and S.286. Retrieved January 21, 2021 from http://www.amhca.org/advocacy/medicare

Bartle-Haring, S., Silverthorn, B. C., Meyer, K., & Toviessi, P. (2009). Does live supervision make a difference? A multilevel analysis. *Journal of Marital and Family Therapy, 35,* 406–414. https://doi.org/10.1111/j.1752-0606.2009.00124.x

Burns, T., & Firn, M. (2017). *Outreach in community mental health care: A manual for practitioners* (2nd ed.). Oxford University Press.

Champe, J., & Kleist, D. M. (2003). Live supervision: A review of the research. *The Family Journal: Counseling and Therapy for Couples and Families, 11,* 268–275. https://doi.org/10.1177/1066480703252755

Cohen, J., Marecek, J., & Gillham, J. (2006). Is three a crowd? Clients, clinicians, and managed care. *American Journal of Orthopsychiatry, 76,* 251–259. https://doi.org/10.1037/e343342004-001

Cooper, C. C., & Gottlieb, M. C. (2000). Ethical issues with managed care: Challenges facing counseling psychology. *The Counseling Psychologist, 28,* 179–236. https://doi.org/10.1177/0011000000282001

Danzinger, P. R., & Welfel, E. R. (2001). The impact of managed care on mental health counselors: A survey of perceptions, practices, and compliance with ethical standards. *Journal of Mental Health Counseling, 23,* 137–150.

Eaves, S., Emens, R., & Sheperis, C. J. (2008). Counselors in the managed care era: The efficacy of the data based problem solver model. *Journal of Professional Counseling: Practice, Theory, & Research, 36*(2), 1–12. https://doi.org/10.1080/15566382.2008.12033845

Lawless, L., Ginter, E., & Kelly, K. (1999). Managed care: What mental health counselors need to know. *Journal of Mental Health Counseling, 21,* 50–65.

Massachusetts Mental Health Counselors Association. (2021). Public Policy Homepage. Retrieved January 21, 2021, from https://www.mamhca.org/public-policy/

National Institute of Mental Health. (2021). NIMH Outreach Partnership Program. Retrieved January 21, 2021, from https://www.nimh.nih.gov/outreach/partnership-program/index.shtml

Rosenberg, E., & DeMaso, D. R. (2008). A doubtful guest: Managed care and mental health. *Child and Adolescent Psychiatric Clinics of North America, 17,* 53–66. https://doi.org/10.1016/j.chc.2007.07.005

Sutton, R. (2015). *The counselor's STEPs for progress notes: A guide to clinical language and documentation* (2nd ed.). CreateSpace Independent Publishing Platform.

Talbott, J. A. (2001). The economics of mental health care in the USA and the potential for managed care to expand into Europe. *Current Opinion in Psychiatry, 14,* 279–285. https://doi.org/10.1097/00001504-200107000-00001

U.S. Department of Health and Human Services. (2021). Health Information Privacy. Retrieved January 21, 2021, from https://www.hhs.gov/hipaa/index.html

Williams, C., Firn, M., Wharne, S., & MacPherson, R. (Eds.). (2011). *Assertive outreach in mental healthcare: Current perspectives.* Wiley-Blackwell.

Wolff, N., & Schlesinger, M. (2002). Clinicians as advocates: An exploratory study of responses to managed care by mental health professionals. *The Journal of Behavioral Health Services and Research, 29,* 274–287. https://doi.org/10.1007/BF02287368

ADDITIONAL RESOURCES

American Foundation for Suicide Prevention website: https://afsp.org/

Anxiety and Depression Association of America website: https://adaa.org/

Banks, B. M. (2018). University mental health outreach targeting students of color. *Journal of College Student Psychotherapy, 34,* 78–86. https://doi.org/10.1080/87568225.2018.1539632

Frank, R. I., & Davidson, J. (2014). *The transdiagnostic road map to case formulation and treatment planning.* New Harbinger.

Haack, L. M., Kapke, T. L., & Gerdes, A. C. (2016). Rates, associations, and predictors of psychopathology in a convenience sample of school-aged Latino youth: Identifying areas for mental health outreach. *Journal of Child and Family Studies, 25,* 2315–2326. https://doi.org/10.1007/s10826-016-0404-y

Lu, C., Frank, R. G., & McGuire, T. G. (2008). Demand response of mental health services to cost sharing under managed care. *Journal of Mental Health Policy and Economics, 11,* 113–125.

MacMillan, T., & Sisselman-Borgia, A. (Eds.). (2018). *New directions in treatment, education, and outreach for mental health addiction.* Springer.

Mental Health America website: https://www.mhanational.org/

Rowe, M., Styron, T., & David, D. H. (2016). Mental health outreach to persons who are homeless: Implications for practice from a statewide study. *Community Mental Health Journal, 52,* 56–65. https://doi.org/10.1007/s10597-015-9963-4

Van Citters, A. D., & Bartels, S. (2004). A systematic review of the effectiveness of community-based mental health outreach services for older adults. *Psychiatric Services, 55,* 1237–1249. https://doi.org/10.1176/appi.ps.55.11.1237

Wilson, H. M. N., Davies, J. S., & Weatherhead, S. (2016). Trainee therapists' experiences of supervision during training: A meta-synthesis. *Clinical Psychology and Psychotherapy, 23,* 340–351. https://doi.org/10.1002/cpp.1957

5

Obtaining the Right Job

■ ■ ■

INTRODUCTION

Your primary goal upon graduation is to find a job as a mental health counselor. The competitiveness of the job market will vary by geographical location, but it is always best to start searching, applying, and (hopefully) interviewing a few months before graduation. Like many students, you probably need employment as soon as possible to start making money and receiving benefits (e.g., health insurance). Also, the sooner you start working, the sooner you can start obtaining postgraduate counseling hours for licensure. You also do not want to put yourself into the position where you are begrudgingly accepting an offer at a not-so-ideal agency because you feel desperate. Preferably, you want to put yourself into a position where you are applying and interviewing at multiple agencies where you have a choice. As clichéd as it sounds, looking for a job is a lot like dating. As much as a potential employer is interviewing you, you should also be interviewing them. You need to do what is best for you when entering a potentially long-term relationship.

The focus of this chapter is not just on finding a job in general; there are many books and chapters available for that. Rather, the focus here is from the perspective of individuals recently graduating with their degree in counseling and looking to get their entry job (or early-career job) as a mental health counselor. Although there is certainly overlap in many of the steps to searching for a job, there are also some nuances to the mental health field that need to be taken into consideration. Through the lens of an early-career counselor, this chapter will cover searching for desirable jobs, developing an appropriate résumé and cover letter, managing your online reputation, and interviewing skills and strategies, including researching agencies and accepting a job offer.

Hopefully, this chapter can provide some guidance and, in the process, reduce some anxiety and boost your confidence. Keep in mind that the person "who gets hired is not necessarily the one who can do that job best; but, the one who knows the most about how to get hired" (Richard Lathrop; as cited in Bolles, 2018, p. 140). Job hunting is both a science and an art. Your first job will most likely not be your job for life, but it is nice to get a good start to your professional career as a mental health counselor at an agency that is nurturing and provides opportunities for growth. Job hunting for your first counselor job should be both enjoyable and rewarding, not stressful and punishing!

SEARCHING FOR DESIRABLE JOBS

You will soon be graduating with your degree in counseling, and you are finally ready to begin looking for your first job as a mental health counselor. Very exciting! What population do you want to work with? What mental health setting do you want to work in? Does agency location matter to you? Do you want to start specializing in a therapeutic approach? What are your salary and benefits expectations? Are you looking for a supervisor with a particular theoretical background? What agency values are most important to you? These are all great questions to consider. However, it is best to initially keep an open mind while doing your job search. Although there may be some positions you have no desire for, you still want to have a wide enough net to keep your options open. There may even be some available positions that do not initially sound attractive, but may later be worth pursuing as you learn more about the job market and your personal interests. With this in mind, where do you begin?

Your first job will not necessarily dictate the rest of your career as a mental health counselor. However, it is helpful to have at least some parameters when you begin your job search. With that said, it is often best to be open to as many job opportunities as possible, as long as you are not compromising your own professional development and mental health. For example, perhaps you know what population you want to work with (e.g., adolescents). This is a good start. More specifically, you would really like to work with adolescent females with eating disorders in a residential facility. This is also good. Nevertheless, there might not be any agencies with an opening for that specific position in your geographic area. Or, perhaps you only apply to the one open position but do not get a job offer. What now? You probably need to be a little more flexible with your job search.

Population and Agency Setting: Start Early with a Wide Net

Be picky… but not too picky. Rather, be picky for the right reasons. Deciding not to apply to an agency because you prefer to work with 14–18-year-olds instead of 18–22-year-olds is probably too picky. Not applying to an agency because it serves the geriatric population and you prefer to work with adolescents and young adults is probably appropriately picky. There may also be other valid reasons, such as an agency with a poor reputation for providing quality supervision to new graduates or an agency that provides minimal vacation time. The point here is that most new graduates are not in the position to be selective to the point where they apply to only one or two agencies; you will be making it difficult for yourself. With that said, you do not want to be applying to agencies where you are almost certain that you will be miserable working there. Although it is great if you find your ideal job, it is also prudent to be willing to compromise. Also, consider that what you may perceive to be your ideal job upon graduation will most likely be much different from your ideal job post-licensure. In summary, have a wide net while also being clear to yourself what filters you use.

As briefly stated earlier, begin your job search as early as a few months before graduation. You probably want to make "real" money sooner than later and you will begin accruing hours toward licensure immediately after graduation. You can even consider applying to attractive job openings if you know you would be able to start working by their start date. (Some agencies will even hire you a few weeks before you graduate if they really want you. You can begin training and acclimating to your environment as you approach your graduation date.) Depending on the geographic region you are applying for jobs, it may be a competitive job market. The sooner you get your name out there, the better chance you have of obtaining a preferred job position.

Before beginning your job search, keep in mind a few qualities of both desired populations you would like to work with and desired agencies you would like to work for (i.e., think filters on your wide net). For populations, perhaps you have a strong preference to work with a specific disorder (or group of disorders). Keep in mind that some disorders lend themselves more to specialization than others. For example, eating disorder or opioid dependency clinics are more common than specialized settings for depression. With that said, specializations are expanding. It is now more common to see specializations in obsessive-compulsive disorder or hoarding, for example. You may also have an age range in mind. Perhaps you really enjoy working with children aged 3–12 and, although you may be fine working with adolescents at times, you prefer not to work with adults (although you will most likely have to, in some fashion, in family therapy). Other population characteristics that may be of interest to you include sexual orientation, socioeconomic status, developed environment (i.e., rural, suburban, or urban), immigrants, veterans, or marginalized populations (e.g., Native Americans, physically disabled). Keep in mind, the particular population you want to work with may be at least partially dictated by the agency setting you want to work in, or vice versa.

For agency settings, consider if you want to work in community mental health (often nonprofit), hospitals, substance abuse treatment centers, corrections facilities, residential/assisted living, K–12 schools, or colleges/universities. (Private practice also can be an option, but generally only once you are independently licensed, and it requires much assistance and forethought—see Chapter 8.) Relatedly, although often implied with some settings, consider options for service delivery: outpatient (may or may not be fee-for-service), intensive outpatient, in-home, partial inpatient, or inpatient. Service delivery is something that can be initially overlooked by many early-career mental health counselors. For example, the type of counseling provided in a traditional outpatient community mental health agency can be dramatically different from an inpatient substance abuse treatment center. You may have some idea of the differences based on your practicum and internship experiences. However, it is always best to talk to other counselors in the field working at these agencies.

Activity 5.1: Population Characteristics and Agency Setting

You are probably more flexible with some of these population characteristics and agency settings than others. Table 5.1 provides a grid for you to consider the interaction of both your desired population characteristics and agency settings. For population, there is also space underneath each characteristic to be more specific (e.g., age range—"adults only"). If desired, you can also provide your weighted level of importance for each characteristic on a 0–10 scale, with zero being absolutely no weight and 10 being greatest weight. Once this is done, use the grid and look at all the possible combinations of population characteristics and agency setting characteristics. Put a happy face into any of the combinations that appear interesting (e.g., age range—adolescents in a residential setting) and even those that are only a little interesting. Also, note that it is common to have multiple population characteristics combined for an agency setting (e.g., veterans with trauma in a hospital setting or immigrant LGBTQ+ adolescents in a community mental health setting). Of course, be careful not to combine too many population characteristics for one agency setting because it can result in too narrow a population that might not be realistic for a job search (two or three combined population qualities is usually the ideal maximum). Also, keep in mind that many agency settings serve a variety of populations unless very specialized. Ideally, have a few population–agency setting combinations (i.e., three or more). Remember, you want to have a wide enough net with a few filters—a balanced level of "pickiness." Feel free to also rank your remaining combinations. You have now made a significant step forward in preparing for your job search.

Table 5.1 Population Characteristics and Agency Setting Grid

Population Characteristics	Agency Setting Characteristics							
	Community Mental Health I:___	Hospital I:___	Substance Abuse Treatment Center I:___	Corrections Facility I:___	Residential/ Assisted Living I:___	K–12 Schools I:___	College/ University I:___	Other I:___
Specific Disorder ___ I:___								
Age Range ___ I:___								
Sexual Orientation ___ I:___								
Socioeconomic Status ___ I:___								
Developed Environment ___ I:___								
Other (e.g., immigrants, veterans, etc.) ___ I:___								

Weighted level of importance (I): 0–10
*Can also note if preferred service delivery is outpatient, intensive outpatient, in-home, partial inpatient, or inpatient.

**Reflection Questions 5.1: Population Characteristics
and Agency Setting Review**

- What population characteristics do you have the greatest interest to work for? What do you find attractive about these population characteristics? How much are you willing to compromise if your ideal population is not readily available?
- What agency settings do you have the greatest interest to work in? What do you find attractive about these agency settings? How much are you willing to compromise if your ideal agency is not readily available?
- What are your population–agency setting combinations? Do any of them appear to you to be attractive job options?
- Are any of your population–agency setting combinations realistic job options in your desired geographic region to work? Are you willing and able to move, if necessary?
- How has this process helped refine your job search (or not)?

The Finer Details of Benefits: Salary Is Important, But It Is Not Everything

You now have a little more focus on possible job options you may be interested in. A part of you might want to skip this discussion and immediately begin your job search and look for positions with the highest salary. Do not do this. First, you may find that many mental health agencies do not provide a salary (or hourly rate) and/or may provide an ambiguous range in their job postings. Second, if you do see a salary in a job posting, it may not be accurate once you sit down and interview (e.g., salary for an entry-level position is typically much less than an experienced licensed position). Third, salary is important, but it truly is not everything. For your own long-term well-being, it is vital to consider many other benefits along with salary.

The quality of a mental health agency as a whole goes beyond salary and benefits. However, while doing your initial job search, you probably do not know too much about the culture and climate of an agency at this point unless you have direct contacts (i.e., networking). Even then, unless an agency clearly has a horrible reputation, you will still want to find out for yourself by at least interviewing if you have a strong interest in a particular position (discussed later). Unfortunately, some agencies also do not share much information about benefits other than "generous benefits package." What does this even mean? Beyond salary, important benefits to consider include health insurance, dental insurance, retirement plan, life insurance, short/long-term disability, extended medical leave, maternity/paternity leave, flexible spending accounts (for medical expenses and/or childcare expenses), tuition/training reimbursement, and vacation days/holidays/personal time off. The following simply highlights what you should expect for benefits from most mental health agencies. Even if you cannot obtain this information during your search, it is still helpful to keep in mind while interviewing and making decisions on job offers.

Salary

To some degree, what to expect for benefits can vary greatly across geographic regions in the United States. Even though salary is not everything, you should still take some time to research the expected average salary for a mental health counselor in your state. A quick search on www.ziprecruiter. com provides average salaries across states. However, be sure to filter your search for an entry-level position (i.e., not licensed mental health counselor) and/or consider the lower end of the average range. Also, keep in mind that salaries can vary greatly within some states (e.g., working in a major city versus a rural town). Another helpful website is www.glassdoor.com, which provides average salaries and ranges, including such filters as company size, years of experience, and specific types of counselors. Glassdoor also allows you to search by name of company and geographic region. This information can be especially helpful if you know the agency and location for particular job postings. With all of this said, keep in mind that websites for salaries may still not be completely accurate because they are often dependent on self-disclosure from other employees in the field. If you have a comfortable relationship with a few recently employed mental health counselors, you can always talk to them. Finally, while doing your job search you can compare notes with your other counselor peers who are also looking for employment. Over time, as you accumulate information, you will have at least a clearer expected salary range.

Health and Dental Insurance

In most circumstances, any full-time job without health insurance should be avoided. In most states, also expect to see most agencies provide dental insurance as well. As with any insurance, the quality of health/dental insurance will vary by plan. ("Mental health" should be included with health, and sometimes vision is included or can be an add-on.) Some agencies also provide multiple options, typically with varying copays and deductibles, depending on the cost of the plan. Additionally, you will need to take into account what percentage of the health/dental insurance cost is covered by the agency. Health insurance is not cheap. The percentage of coverage should be considered within the context of salary. The point here is that it is good to know if a potential employer provides health/dental insurance, but it is okay to ask for additional details. Most agencies can provide a 1–2-page quick fact sheet explaining their health and dental plans.

Retirement Plan
No matter your age, always take advantage of an employer offering a retirement plan. If a retirement plan is offered, it will most likely be a 401(k) or a 403(b). Typically, nonprofit agencies offer a 403(b) and for-profit agencies offer a 401(k). However, nonprofit agencies can also choose to offer a 401(k). What you should know is that these retirement plans allow you to take out money based on a percentage of your base salary before each paycheck, pretax (this is good for you), which is then invested into mutual funds (401[k] and 403[b]), annuity contracts (401[k] only), and individually managed portfolios (401[k] only). There are other minor differences between a 401(k) and 403(b), but they are well beyond the scope of this book and will most likely not be a deciding factor choosing an agency to work for. The aggressiveness or conservativeness of your retirement plan can be based upon your current age and planned retirement age or customized to your own personal approach. You may even find an agency that will "match" a portion of your contribution (up to a maximum percentage). Whenever possible, do your best to contribute up to the maximum percentage that the agency matches. For example, perhaps an agency matches 50% of what you contribute to your retirement plan up to 5%. This means that if you contribute $100 every period (5% of your salary) the agency will contribute another $50. This is excellent for you! It is free money—how rare is that? Get the most for your money. A final tip is to begin your retirement plan as soon as allowed by the agency. Not only does it start you early with your retirement plan, it also lets you get comfortable living with the amount of money from your paycheck. If you do not start with a retirement plan, you might find it hard if you see less money in your paycheck after the fact.

Safety Net Options
Additional nice "safety net" benefits include life insurance, short/long-term disability, extended medical leave, and maternity/paternity leave. Although these are seemingly morbid thoughts, especially if you are relatively young, it does not hurt to consider the potential of becoming seriously injured or sick. Disability provides you a portion of your income if you are unable to work. Even life insurance is a good option, especially if you have other people's lives you are responsible for (e.g., spouse, children, parents). These benefits are often at minimal cost to you if obtained through your agency. It is best to take advantage of them regardless of age and current health.

Flexible Spending Accounts

Flexible spending accounts (FSAs) are for medical and dependent care expenses. These accounts allow you to set aside a specified amount of money each fiscal year into a separate account for you to use at a later date. This money is then taken out of each paycheck, pretax. It is nice to have some saved-up money in your medical FSA for an unexpected emergency copay, for example. Also, if you have children, then you probably already know that childcare is not cheap. It can be very helpful to have that money put aside to use strictly for dependent care services. What is good about FSAs is that you can save some money to use on medical/dependent care expenses because it is not taxed. Also, you can treat this as a separate savings account where you are not expecting to see the money in your paycheck (like your retirement plan). Keep in mind that there is a caveat to each FSA. For medical FSA, there may be a certain amount that you have to spend by the end of the fiscal year or you lose the money. For example, many FSAs let you roll over up to $500 each fiscal year. Thus, if you took out $750 for the fiscal year, you need to make sure you spend at least $250 before the next fiscal year or anything over $500 is lost. The dependent care FSA is less forgiving. You have to spend all of the money by the fiscal year or you lose whatever is left, whether it is $10 or $1000. Needless to say, the dependent care FSA requires some planning ahead.

Tuition and Training Reimbursement

Take advantage of any tuition or training reimbursement benefits. Even though you already have a graduate degree, you may want to someday obtain a certificate in a specialized area or perhaps you would like to take an occasional graduate course to stay active with current treatments/interventions. Many times, agencies will reimburse a certain percentage or amount for tuition each fiscal year. Your agency might even have a special tuition reimbursement plan with local colleges/universities. Training reimbursement is something that you will definitely use, as all states require continuing education units/credits (CEUs) once you get licensed (CEUs are discussed in Chapter 7). CEUs demonstrate that you are staying up-to-date with the counseling field (e.g., interventions, ethics, supervision). Depending on the state you are licensed in, you will be required to obtain a specific number of CEUs to keep your license active. These trainings are often not cheap ($50–100 per CEU). It is a great option to get reimbursed for required trainings, even if partial.

Time Off

Lastly, strongly consider how much time you get off each year. Each agency varies in how they provide time off to their employees. At the very least, consider how many and what holidays you get off. (You may also want to consider if you have to work weekends and/or early mornings or late nights.) Obviously, you want to have vacation time. Many agencies also now provide mental health and/or personal days. It is hard to say what you should expect for total time off because (again) this can vary greatly by state and the system used for time off. Many agencies are now using what is called personal time off (PTO), which is a total accrual of hours that can be used for vacation days/holidays/personal days. This typically works by adding hours to your "PTO bank" each paycheck. If you are looking at multiple agencies that use PTO, assuming everything else is equal, you might be able to compare their accrual rates (e.g., 7.50 hours every two weeks vs. 8.0 hours every two weeks). Typically, these accrual rates will increase over time as you continue to work for the agency (i.e., more PTO).

Overall, there is a lot to consider with benefits beyond salary. Again, your job search may yield some of this information, while other information will not be obtained until you begin your interview (unless you know someone on the "inside"). Do your best to consider the full impact of all these benefits within the context of the salary, the cost of living, and available resources where you will be living and working. Consider: Job A pays five thousand dollars more in yearly salary than Job B. However, Job B provides better health insurance (quality and cost), has a retirement plan with an agency match (Job B has no match), provides more money in CEU reimbursement, and gives two more weeks of PTO. Job B is probably a much better choice. In fact, if you include the value of the benefits, Job B probably results in more actual money in your pocket now and in the future.

Reflection Questions 5.2: Considering the Benefits of Benefits

- How flexible are you willing to be with salary while considering the availability of other benefits?
- What are your thoughts about immediately contributing to a retirement plan once hired?
- How important is it to you to receive tuition and training reimbursement once you already have completed your graduate degree?
- How much do you value PTO considering the nature of the mental health field (see Chapter 6 on self-care and burnout)?

The Job Search

Now that you have a little more clarity on the type of job you want to search for and some background knowledge about benefits, you are ready to start looking for a job! Where to start? You are most likely thinking, "the Internet," and you are correct, in part. Using the Internet can include a few strategies such as job searching services, websites of specific agencies, and job/agency review services. There is much information out there that is relatively easily accessible. The true skill is knowing how to filter all that information. What can sometimes get overlooked, but is often more effective than internet strategies in some instances, is networking. Who you know, and how you utilize those you know, can greatly enhance your job search. Naturally, it is also important to understand as much information as possible about a job posting when making your decision to apply.

Use the Internet

There are many search engines available to search for mental health counselor jobs. A simple internet search for "job search" will result in many great websites. Some of the more common search websites for counselor jobs include www.indeed.com, www.careerbuilder.com, www.ziprecruiter.com, www.monster.com, and www.glassdoor.com. It is impossible to suggest one job search website over another because it really depends on what websites the mental health agencies in your geographic area prefer to use. Some agencies use just one website, others use multiple websites. It is best to use as many websites as possible so that your job search is as thorough as possible. If you are not finding enough jobs with the above-noted websites, then search the Internet for additional job search websites.

Although each job search website may have its own unique features, they have many common features (or filters) as well: job title, location (city/town and state), job type (e.g., full-time, part-time, contract), salary, experience level (e.g., entry, mid, senior), and agency name. In your case, because you are searching for your first job as a mental health counselor, it is best to minimize the filters you use unless you are getting more than a few hundred jobs per search. It is highly recommended to start with job title and location (within your desired radius) and then adjust any of the filters from there, if necessary.

Your search will most likely yield many hits, but not all of them may be relevant to what you are looking for. In some cases, you might be able to screen out certain job postings based on the title. Other times, you will need to click on the title to read the job description. A good job description will first describe the agency (including website, populations served, agency values, and/or mission statement) and responsibilities. There should be additional information such as full-time/part-time, salary (or hourly rate), benefits, required education level, required experience level (often based on years or licensure), and required license. You will then have the option to apply through the job search website or the agency. What is often required for the initial application is some general/basic background information and a résumé. (Additional information such as graduate transcripts, references, and criminal background check often comes later if you are asked to interview.) An agency may also request a cover letter. It is suggested to always provide a cover letter with your résumé even if not requested. (The next section addresses résumé and cover letter development.)

An important caveat to address when doing an internet job search is to be aware of how particular words or phrases affect the search. Keep this in mind if you find that your search results in many jobs not related to counseling or in a different profession. This sounds obvious, but it is especially important because of the generic use of the word "counselor." For example, there are many other position titles in the mental health field that use the word counselor: "residential counselor," "classroom counselor," or "support counselor." You will notice that most of these positions (often bachelor's level or less) are not relevant to your level of education. There are also other professions that use the word counselor: "guidance counselor," "rehabilitation counselor," or "spiritual counselor." These positions are probably not directly related to your training.

If you are getting too many false hits due to using the word counselor, consider expanding your search with a few additional words in quotes. For example, simply using "mental health counselor" or "clinical professional counselor" can result in a more refined and accurate search. Also, the mental health field often uses other words besides counselor that are synonymous, such as "therapist" or "clinician." Substituting counselor with therapist and clinician and using a few additional words can result in a greater proportion of desired job positions than of false hits. Over time, you will become familiar with the most appropriate words or phrases. Additionally, do your best to learn the language commonly used within your state. You can easily pick up on this during your practicum/internship and in your advanced courses. Simply listen to how your colleagues and professors talk when referring to themselves or other mental health counselors. Of course, you can always simply ask!

Finally, you can also directly search for job postings at agency websites. Some agencies have their own portal to submit an application. Other agencies have job postings but have a link that will redirect you to a job search website. Whenever possible, submit your application directly through the agency website. You may be given a person's name as a direct contact during your submission, and you can be more confident that your application is received. In general, it is a good habit to become familiar with the content of agency websites because not only will this information help you tailor your résumé and cover letter, it can also be used to prepare for an interview (discussed later in this chapter).

Initially, you may not know of any agencies in your desired geographic region. However, while doing your job search, you will quickly learn what agencies are looking for counselors. Furthermore, if you are looking in the same area as your internship/practicum, you already know of at least one agency and have probably learned of a few others during your interactions with other colleagues. Your peers in your practicum/internship course have placements different from your own. You can also ask the professors in your program, as they are probably well networked within the field. Sometimes your networked contacts can lead you directly to the source and bypass the internet job search.

Network, Then Network Some More

A good tip in life is never to burn your bridges, unless it is really necessary. The best way to not burn bridges is to treat others with dignity and respect (like your clients!) and maintain some form of contact, whenever possible (LinkedIn is a good source—discussed in the "Managing Your Online Reputation" section later). Specific to the counseling profession, the relationships you establish from your first day of graduate school onward may have professional benefits in the years ahead, in many ways that you cannot foresee. Point being, your professors, practicum/internship supervisors and colleagues, research mentors, and even your own peers could someday help you land your first (and future) counseling job. This is especially true if you plan on obtaining your first job within the same geographic region as your graduate program.

If you do not burn your bridges, you will be able to develop "bridge-people" over time (you will become one for others, too). These bridge-people might be able to someday help you connect with others within the counseling profession. This is called networking. The more bridge-people you have in your professional life, the larger your network (think of a spider web growing in size). Many counseling professionals obtain their jobs through networking. Sometimes, it is about who you know. For example, perhaps one of the professors in your graduate program keeps in contact with senior alumni who are now administrators at multiple agencies within the region. In fact, some of these alumni ask this professor to refer quality counseling students in your program to their agency (perhaps some "home team" preference). This professor may then be privy to early information about new job postings within these agencies and pass them on to you and some of your fellow peers. If you have a good relationship with this professor, you could also use this individual as a professional reference. In this case, not only are you applying early for a potentially competitive job position, but you also have an "in" because your professor is willing to speak positively about you. Furthermore, the hiring individuals at the agency greatly value your graduate program and your professor's words/opinion. Of course, you will still have to interview along with other qualified candidates. There is still no guarantee that you will get the job, but you would most likely be a few steps ahead of other candidates. Also, if you are really lucky, you could land a job early in your job search and not have to spend much time job searching on the Internet.

A final social caveat about networking is simply to be careful about what you say in front of whom. In other words, while you are trying to network yourself, keep in mind that your professors, practicum/internship supervisors, and colleagues are most likely very well networked. Think of the six degrees of Kevin Bacon, which posits that any two people on Earth are six or fewer acquaintance links apart. In the mental health field, look at it as three degrees of "put name of professor or supervisor here" within your geographic region. Point being, even though you may say something negative about an individual/agency and she/he/it is not present, somebody else might be present who knows that individual/agency. People talk. It could even be a peer, with no malicious intent, who shares what you said to others. If you find that you are a very talkative person, simply follow some old advice: "If you don't have something nice to say, don't say anything at all." This also holds true for your social media accounts. You do not want to inadvertently burn a bridge that could be helpful in the future.

Things You Should Know about the Job Position
In order to ensure that you are applying for an appropriate job position, pay close attention not only to the job description, but also to the required level of education and experience. The mental health field has a variety of available positions ranging from bachelor's level to doctoral level. You might see a title like "residential counselor." However, after you read the description you may realize it is not a position that provides counseling (or therapy) for clients. Rather, it is a direct-care staff that interacts with the clients within the milieu, typically a bachelor's level position. There may even be some job descriptions that appear to provide counseling to clients, but you notice that the required education is "bachelor's or higher." You technically do qualify for this position, but you may find yourself working in an environment with those much less trained than you and probably not providing "true counseling" (e.g., daily check-ins and not addressing true mental health issues). This can result in a negative experience. On top of that, your salary will probably not match your level of education.

Experience can refer to years working in the filed or whether you have your license or not. In most cases, agencies will note if the job position is for a licensed or prelicensed mental health counselor. This is an important distinction. If the job posting clearly states a license is required, then you should not apply for this position. As discussed in Chapter 3, some states have different levels of licensure. If that is the case, take note of the specific level of licensure stated in the description. You need to make sure that you meet that licensure level or higher. You will find jobs that state "license-eligible" or "prelicensure" (or even state "entry level"). These positions clearly apply to you. Some agencies are looking to hire entry-level counselors like yourself. Finally, you may notice that some postings state "license preferred." Many early-career counselors will avoid applying because they think they do not have a chance. However, sometimes this is not the case. An agency would not post this requirement if there was no interest in a non-licensed counselor. You never know whether you will get an interview unless you apply.

There are a few other things to take into consideration if provided in the job description. Hopefully, at the very least, job duties will be described. Some job positions have really great titles, but what the actual duties entail could greatly vary from what you envision. Be sure that the job duties match your level of education and involve providing face-to-face counseling. There are the occasional job postings that state "master's required," but upon further review you may notice the job requires little to no counseling skills. Not only do you want a job that allows you to develop your counseling skills (what you went to graduate school for!), but you also need client counseling hours for your eventual license. Relatedly, check to see if supervision is provided for early-career counselors and, if so, whether it will be by an approved supervisor as defined by your state and will be on or off site. Unfortunately, not all agencies provide this information in their posted job descriptions. These would definitely be questions to ask if you apply and are offered an interview.

A final comment should be made here about fee-for-service positions. A fee-for-service counselor gets paid based on number of clients billed each week. There are many models of fee-for-service counseling/billing. Some agency fee-for-service models work well due to their flexibility and availability of benefits. However, be leery of any agency fee-for-service model that does not immediately provide benefits or the benefits are strictly contingent on billable hours. What this means is that you either do not get benefits or, if you do, you may lose your benefits if you do not keep up with the billable hours. Some agencies do this to save revenue. This is usually not a good system, especially for beginning counselors. The last thing you want to be worrying about while working toward licensure is making sure you have enough billable hours in order to continue receiving benefits. This is also a good example of not just focusing on the salary. You may be initially enticed by such models because you notice what you would get paid per billable hour. Yet, keep in mind how much you take home after taxes and how much you will be paying out of pocket for benefits not provided (e.g., medical and/or dental) and money not being saved for the future (e.g., retirement plan). What used to be a high-salary position may now be one of the lowest-salary positions. Again, fee-for-serve job descriptions may not provide many details. You will need to follow up with more questions during your interview if you choose to apply.

Reflection Questions 5.3: Job Search Preparation Thoughts

- How confident are you in your internet skills to search for job positions? Do you have any potential concerns using the Internet for job searching, even if skilled?
- What are your thoughts about using networking as the primary method for job searching?
- Do you think you have the contacts necessary for effective networking? What have you done/can you do to develop a network for job searching?
- What are your thoughts about applying for a job position that states "licensed preferred"?

Activity 5.2: Job Search: Making a List and Checking It Twice (and Many More Times)

A lot of the information to consider during a job search has been reviewed. For most people it is helpful to use a table to organize all this information, including agency and job comparison along with planning ahead. Table 5.2 is a job search table that provides multiple categories to consider for each job position. First, for each row there is room to list the job title and provide a brief description. Second, there are columns available to provide a variety of information for each job position beginning with agency information: name (contact, if provided), location, setting, and population. You can also note any salary and benefits information, if provided. It is important to note licensure, if eligible or required. Even if a job is "license required," still consider including it in your table if you find it very attractive. You might refer back to this table in the future. If desired, there is additional space to note if you submitted your résumé/cover letter, have begun researching the agency (discussed later), and received an interview offer/date. Of course, you will want to use a separate form for listing strengths and weaknesses (see Table 5.4 discussed later). Putting some brief thoughts in the table will allow for comparison with other agencies/job positions.

Table 5.2   Job Search Table

| | Agency | | | Salary | Benefits Provided | Licensure (Eligible or Required) | Submit Résumé/ CL? | Agency Researched? | Interview Offer & Date |
	Name & Contact	Location	Setting & Population						
1. Job Title _____ Description _____ _____ _____									
2. Job Title _____ Description _____ _____ _____									
3. Job Title _____ Description _____ _____ _____									

Reflection Questions 5.4: Job Search Review

- Were you able to find a satisfactory number of job positions that serve your desired client characteristics and agency setting characteristics? What are your thoughts on what is available?
- Did you find any job positions interesting (maybe even worth applying for) that you did not expect? What makes these job positions interesting/attractive?
- Identify at least two job positions that you actually would seriously consider applying for. What are your reasons for selecting these job positions?
- Discuss your thoughts and feelings about this job search experience. What did you learn? Do you feel more (or less) optimistic about obtaining a job upon graduation? How do you plan on moving forward?

RÉSUMÉ AND COVER LETTER

When applying for a job position, the mental health agency may have you fill out a form with additional background details. It is rare to see requests for additional information demonstrating counseling skills before the interview (e.g., short-answer questions). Thus, your application is essentially your résumé and cover letter. Unless you have used your social networks, this is all the information hiring agencies will know about you, so make it good. If you get to the interview stage, you can "show" yourself more and most likely share your references (rarely looked at before the interview); but first show the best of yourself in the best way on paper (or electronic paper). Much time and thought should be put into developing your résumé and cover letter. Even if you already have a résumé and experience writing a cover letter, the following information should still be helpful in tailoring these documents specifically to the mental health profession.

Résumé

You are probably more than familiar with what is a résumé and its purpose. You possibly needed to submit one to get into undergraduate and graduate school, or any jobs or internships you have had up to this point. In general, a résumé is a summary of your educational and professional qualifications and experiences. At this point in your career, your résumé's primary purpose is a key part of your job application. You have also probably heard of many suggestions (e.g., "do's" and "don'ts") for résumé writing. Many times, these suggestions come from the business field. Some of the business field suggestions are still appropriate to the counseling profession, while others are not applicable. The goal here is to provide guidance in developing a résumé that puts you in a good position when applying for mental health counselor jobs. Lastly, your résumé should be a working document, something that is frequently revised. It can be difficult to remember particular details of certain experiences over time. Do your best to revise and update your résumé at least every 3–4 months. Even if you are sure you have nothing to add, still take the time to read it over to make sure everything still looks appropriate.

If you have not figured it out yet, your résumé is very important when applying for jobs. Your résumé and cover letter (discussed next) are often the only two documents a potential employer will look at. On top of that, they may be looked at for only a few seconds or minutes. How much attention your résumé receives truly depends on the agency and number of applicants. If you have key words and desired experiences that get the attention of the person reviewing your application, it will be given more time and consideration. In the business world, many times your application is thoroughly prescreened by human resources before it moves on to the appropriate department. Although this can certainly happen in the mental health field, many times your application goes straight to those who will be directly hiring you (and supervising you), possibly after a brief screening by human resources to ensure basic minimum requirements are met. (In fact, sometimes you might email your application materials directly to a potential supervisor, for example.)

Furthermore, those reviewing your application are looking not only for desired skills and qualities but also for anything that might stick out to disqualify you. Look at it this way: screening résumés is much more time- and money-efficient than face-to-face interviews. Not everybody who applies for a job position will receive an interview. It is not practical. Thus, for both your résumé and cover letter, do your best to highlight your qualifications without trying too hard by sharing too much information, highlighting your weaknesses, and/or making spelling/formatting mistakes. If it helps you conceptualize the purpose of your résumé, look at it from the perspective of getting to the next step—the interview. At this point, you are not selling yourself to secure a job; you want to get invited for an interview. Face-to-face interactions are where you can sell yourself, not through your résumé. This approach reduces the chances that you will be screened out for any red flags or awkward content. At this point, you just need to get your foot inside the door.

Basics

You may also have heard of a curriculum vitae (CV), especially as a student interacting with your professors. Perhaps you developed something like this to apply to graduate school. In Latin, curriculum vitae means "course of life." An oversimplified definition of CV is a very detailed résumé. For academics, a CV not only highlights educational and professional qualifications and experiences, but it also greatly focuses on service to the college/ university (including community) and research-related accomplishments (e.g., publications and conference presentations). The résumé format proposed here is like a hybrid of a résumé and a CV. In general, a résumé–CV hybrid allows for greater detail in describing your relevant experiences (e.g., work, volunteering, or counseling), whereas a typical résumé is very brief in describing experiences (and very brief in general). On the other hand, your résumé–CV hybrid will still be succinct enough to highlight key experiences without getting bogged down in the minute details.

You are probably now thinking, "how long should this 'résumé–CV' document be?" The answer is, "not too long, but not too short." Ha! A very common "old-school" suggestion for résumés is no more than one page. This may still be true in some parts of the business world, but it does not realistically apply to professional counseling. Our field generally does not have physical, measurable outputs (e.g., 10 widgets made per day or developed marketing portfolio to save $10,000 a quarter) unless you are in an upper administration position. Our field serves individuals experiencing mental health distress, which requires more description to provide context (i.e., cannot be put into numbers). When describing each of your experiences, be detailed, using bullet points (or a similar approach) to highlight your relevant skills. In most cases a résumé can be two to three pages, possibly even four if you have extensive professional/life experience. Two to three pages is often considered the "sweet spot" because it allows just enough room to highlight particular job experiences while not being too detailed with information that would better be integrated into your cover letter or completely left out.

Before getting into the actual content of a résumé, it is important to address formatting. Although it may sound superficial, make sure that your résumé looks "nice" on the surface. After giving an initial positive impression, your résumé may get a closer look. Nothing can be more of a turnoff to a potential employer than a résumé that shows inconsistent format size, poor spacing, or disorganized headings. If you cannot look good on paper, why would they assume you would look good in person? Keep in mind that there are no set rules on how to format a résumé. You may have a unique style that works for you. The following are some general "safe" suggestions. First, use a 12–14-point font size and a professional/business font style (e.g., Times New Roman or Arial). (Also, avoid trying too hard with a cursive font like Lucida Calligraphy [even though it does look cool].) Using a font style like Comic Sans MS or Herculanum does not exactly communicate professionalism. You want the people reviewing your résumé to actually see and understand the content of your résumé (and not laugh at you!). Having headers and subheadings that are centered and/or aligned left in bold and/or underlined helps make your major sections and subsections stand out for quick scans. (Also, do not use a heading at the end of one page with no content until the next page. It looks weird. Move the heading to the next page.) When entering the content for each of your headings, it is generally preferred that your most recent experiences and accomplishments be listed first (i.e., on top) followed chronologically by older ones (e.g., current job from 2021 to present is listed first, previous job from 2019–2020 listed next/below).

Whenever possible, do your best to write in active voice instead of passive voice. Typically, passive-voice sentences use more words and can be vague. Also, passive voice can come off a bit boring and indirectly does not give you as much credit for the particular activity. With active voice, the subject of the sentence performs the action (e.g., [I] completed intakes with adolescents and their families.). With passive voice the subject receives the action (e.g., Intakes with adolescents and their families were completed [by me]). A quick way to tell if you are using active or passive voice is to add "by zombies" (or any silly statement) to the end of the sentence. If the sentence still makes sense with the addition (e.g., "Intakes with adolescents and their families were completed by zombies."), then it is passive. Always avoid zombies.

It should go without saying to make sure there are no grammar or spelling errors. This can be a major turnoff for most résumé reviewers. You might be able to get away with a minor mistake (or even two), but any more and your chances of being asked for an interview are nil. This means, do not just rely on the spellcheck function in your word processing program. Not all typos, spelling/grammar errors, and awkward phrases are picked up by such programs. Reread and revise your résumé a few days after completing a draft (i.e., put it down and come back later). Relatedly, avoid lazy writing ("e.g.," "etc.," or "same as above")—write it out! Ideally, also have a trusted friend, colleague, or even a professor look it over. In the end, regardless of your style, just make sure the document looks well organized and is easy to follow. In other words, do not frustrate the person reviewing your résumé.

Key Content

Part of making your résumé attractive to reviewers is including the right content (i.e., headings) organized in an appropriate order. There is no perfect way to organize the content of your résumé, but some styles can be a turnoff to reviewers (e.g., listing your education at the end of the résumé).

Regardless of style, do your best to include any relevant and appropriate experiences from your undergraduate years onward. Typically, experiences/accomplishments while in high school are not included unless they are something of great significance. Remember, mental health agencies are not just looking at your most recent past experiences; they want to see the bigger picture as well.

The first thing that should go on your résumé is your name and additional identifying/contact information. Whenever possible, it is strongly suggested to leave out your home address and personal phone number, especially if posting to a public website (e.g., a job search website or LinkedIn). It is all too easy for your information to become available on the Internet. You can always include this information in your cover letter, which is generally not posted on the Internet. You can also consider including just the town and state you live in and provide a work phone number. (If you really want to include such personal information, you could always create two versions: one for public posting, and one for direct submission to agencies.) If you do include a phone number, make sure your voicemail is your own (i.e., not shared with a friend or family member) and appropriate (e.g., no intro music of "Who Let the Dogs Out"). You can include your email address. If available, provide a professional (e.g., internship) or academic email address. However, keep in mind that you might not have access to these email addresses or work phone numbers after graduation. It is fine to use your own personal email address, just make sure it is appropriate. A reviewer seeing an email address like "keg_master@" or "crazy4pot@" is probably going to skip over that résumé very quickly. Also feel free to include any professional profiles you may have like your LinkedIn link or a personal website. Of course, make sure that the content of these sources is appropriate. Additionally, do not share your gender (although sometimes obvious based on your name), age, race/ethnicity, religion, sexual orientation, relationship status, or any other personal or physical characteristics. It should also go without saying to not include your marital status, number of children, current salary, or hobbies. Finally, in case you were considering including a personal photo—do not. Save that for your LinkedIn profile.

The next section of your résumé should be "Education," which includes your bachelor's degree and master's degree. You can either provide the letters for your degree (e.g., B.S. or M.A.) or spell it out (e.g., Master of Arts; note it is not "Master's" of Arts—no possessive) and then state your major (e.g., Psychology) and any minors. Of course, include the college/university, including date of graduation (anticipated date provided if not yet graduated). Also include any concentrations you may have completed while in graduate school (e.g., Cognitive-Behavioral Therapies or Child and Family Interventions) and the title of any completed theses. It is your choice if you want to provide your grade point average (GPA) or class rank. If it is below 3.0 for undergraduate and below 3.5 for graduate, you may not want to include it (may hurt more than help). You can also state your "laude" status (e.g., Cum Laude, Magna Cum Laude, or Summa Cum Laude). Finally, do not list coursework. If you specialized in a particular area you will most likely have a concentration or certification to list; that is enough. If a potential employer really wants to know what courses you took, they can review your transcript during the interview stage.

A section that some like to put soon after Education is "Honors or Awards." Some prefer to also put this toward the end of their résumé; either way can work. If you do have any honors or awards, do not be hesitant to list them. Provide the name of the award and the year and month it was received. It is also strongly suggested to provide a brief description for each award if the title is not clear on what it was for (assume most people are not familiar with the award[s] you received).

Another section that can go soon after Education or toward the end of your résumé is "Professional Affiliations." Although you are early in your career, you might already be a member of the American Counseling Association (ACA) or the American Mental Health Counselors Association (AMHCA), for example. You can also identify any affiliations you obtained while an undergraduate (e.g., Psi Chi—The International Honor Society of Psychology). It is appropriate to list any professional association you may have that is related to clinical mental health counseling or other academic societies (e.g., perhaps you are part of the Spanish National Honor Society). You may have even received a local, state, or national award for excellence in service to the community. These affiliations show your dedication to the field of counseling, academics, and the community.

Your next section should be "Counseling/Clinical Experience" or some other similar title that reflects clinical mental health counseling experience. Admittedly, this section might not have many job positions to list. However, at the very least you will have your practicum and internship experiences to include. You may have also had a part-time job while in school and/or an undergraduate internship that included working in the mental health field (e.g., an assistant to an applied behavioral analysis [ABA] specialist working with those with autism). This is a section where it is important to be more detailed with your duties because this shows how you have applied your counseling skills in your early professional career. Examples to include are intakes, assessments administered and scored, case formulations and treatment plans, examples of interventions (possibly emphasizing a theoretical orientation), participating in team meetings, types of therapy modality provided (e.g., individual, family, group), description of the setting, and population served. Be sure to include the agency's name (provide city and state as well), title of your position, and date range of employment. It is also suggested that you provide the full name of any of your supervisors, including their license and any other relevant credentials. Try not to feel too distressed if you provide only one or two positions in this section. It is okay. Agencies looking for early-career counselors understand that you have been in the field for only a few years, at most. Just do your best to highlight your experience up to this point.

Another section to include is "Work Experience." This can include any other job positions you have had that are not related to clinical mental health counseling. Having other jobs demonstrates the ability to handle responsibilities and a level of professionalism. Also, you might have had some jobs in the past that have transferrable skills (e.g., summer camp residential counselor). The recommendations for "Clinical/Counseling Experience" content should be followed here as well, especially if you think that you had some responsibilities that overlap with counseling. One caveat here is to avoid listing any unrelated jobs that may have a negative perception (fair or not). For example, highlighting your duties at "Bob's Slick Car Sales" might not be the best choice.

A similar section to "Clinical/Counseling Experience" and "Work Experience" is "Volunteer Work." As the name states, this includes any service you have provided to others or the community that did not include any formal pay. There is a good chance you have participated in a few volunteer activities that have some skills transferable to counseling (e.g., Big Brother/Big Sister). Dedicating your time to helping others without pay can be an attractive quality to some agencies.

Toward the end of your résumé you can list any other relevant experiences that may be attractive to agencies. One common area for some graduate students is "Research Experience." Here, you can you list the research team (including professor, for example) that worked for, the focus of the research, and your specific duties. You may even have presented at a professional conference or gotten your name on a peer-reviewed journal article. Definitely include such accomplishments. On the other hand, it is best to not list any conferences attended if you did not present.

A common section toward the end of the résumé is "Other Relevant Skills" or a similar title. This is where you can list any other skills you have that might be relevant/attractive to a mental health agency. Examples include another language besides English (being bilingual—or more—can be an attractive quality), knowledge of computer programs or internet skills beyond the basics (e.g., statistics, web design), and certifications (e.g., CPR, first aid, crisis management).

The most common final section of a résumé is "References." It is now becoming less common to include a References section. That is also the suggestion here. It is also not worthwhile to include a References section and then state "available upon request." Doing this really serves no purpose (of course, references should always be available upon request!). Although some may disagree with this suggestion, many mental health professionals who hire candidates believe it is more appropriate to request references from a prospective employee after they have had a chance to interview you. In almost all cases, a mental health agency reviewing your application is not going to contact your references until after an interview. It is more efficient with their time to screen you in/out with your résumé and cover letter and then get a face-to-face impression of you before making phone calls, which can take considerably more time than you may think (e.g., phone tag setting up a time to talk, asking semi-structured questions). Also, your references might not want their contact information being distributed across the Internet. Thus, if your interview goes well, you will most likely be asked to provide a list of references. This is when you can hand them (or email) a separate document with your references. Even in the unusual circumstance where an agency requests your references before your interview, you can always provide this document. An ideal number is three references. Some agencies might be okay with two, but always having at least three on hand is the safest option. Your reference list should include, name, title, institution, and contact information, including a phone number for a verbal reference. You can include their role in their relationship with you (e.g., professor, counseling supervisor). There may be circumstances where you have a pre-written reference available to provide (e.g., professor is retiring).

Do make sure you receive permission from those you want to include as a reference. Not only is it the respectful and professional thing to do, it is also for your own benefit. In most cases, you probably have a good enough relationship with these individuals in the first place to even be asking. However, you do not want to make any assumptions. Have a meeting with these individuals to ask them if they are both willing to be a reference and if they can be positive and supportive. Most individuals will be honest with you. Very few will agree to be a reference and then say negative things about you (this would not be cool!). Your references should include professionals in the field that can attest to your counseling knowledge and skills and your interpersonal skills. You will most likely be asking professors and practicum/internship instructors and supervisors. You may also have a supervisor at your current job who could be a good reference. It should go without saying that you should not include your significant other, family members, friends, or your own counselor as references!

You may have noticed that no "Objective" section was recommended. This part of the résumé does not serve much purpose in modern job applications, especially if you are providing a cover letter. Often the objective statement is generic: "to obtain a job as a mental health counselor." No kidding, you just applied. It may also include generic personal quality statements: "I am hardworking, willing to learn, and a team player." This is nice, but it does not really say anything unique about you. Who would not say this about themselves?

Finally, if you want to submit a paper version of your résumé and are thinking about laminating it . . . do not. It is not cool.

Cover Letter

A cover letter is a short document that allows you to introduce yourself on a personal level while connecting to a specific agency based on your professional skills and experiences and your personal attributes. Even if not requested in a job position, it is usually a good idea to submit a cover letter with your résumé. A great cover letter can make a strong first impression. Keep this in mind if you are still feeling a little insecure about the "substance" of your résumé. A cover letter is a good way to enhance your professional and personal strengths. You can also include information that would not be appropriate or practical to include in your résumé. If done wisely, a cover letter can help the people reviewing your application to connect the parts of your résumé that are the most relevant for the job you are applying for.

Although it can be helpful to modify your résumé for each job position, your cover letter should truly be unique and specific for each job position you apply for. In other words, avoid a cookie-cutter cover letter where you just change the name of the job position and agency. This means, take the time to further research the agency, not just the specific job position. Try to get a sense of the populations they serve, their approach to counseling (e.g., emphasize use of evidenced-based interventions with interpersonal approaches), desired qualifications for your position, and their overall agency values (e.g., see mission statement). When possible, it is helpful to integrate key words into your cover letter to match the job description/ requirements and the agency itself. This includes highlighting relevant accomplishments on your résumé, such as education, counseling, and/or research experiences that match the job. However, make sure you do not regurgitate your résumé. Your cover letter should not be a summary of your résumé. It should provide relevant context for your résumé in relation to the job position. Overall, similar to earlier comments about your résumé, the purpose of your cover letter is to help you get an interview. Highlight your strengths and qualifications without sharing too much personal information, especially your weaknesses. Save the more personal information (still judiciously) for the interview.

Basics

The length of your cover letter should generally be no more than one page, but going a little over onto a second page is usually fine. Three or more pages is definitely not recommended. A cover letter is typically single spaced with block paragraphs. Your formatting should be the same as your résumé: 12–14 point font size and a professional/business font style (consider matching your résumé). Be sure to write in an active voice instead of a passive voice. Do your best to also downplay the use of adverbs (e.g., "extremely excited for the opportunity to work for such a super amazing company" or "very eagerly applying for your wicked neat job position"). Overuse of adverbs can come off as dramatic (and in turn, insincere) and immature. Also have your cover letter reviewed not just for grammar/spelling errors and lazy writing ("e.g.," "etc.," or "same as above") like your résumé, but also for appropriateness of content and overall flow. You might want to consider giving a brief job and agency description to the individual reviewing your cover letter. There is also a great application that can provide feedback on how well your sentences read: www.hemingwayapp.com. Remember, your cover letter will be more personalized and specific to the job position. Simply having good formatting and grammar/spelling might not be enough.

Key Content
Before even writing your cover letter, be sure to use the correct agency name in the address line and hiring manager/supervisor/contact in your greeting (and throughout the cover letter). This is a common mistake made when applying to many positions while using one cover letter as a template for multiple cover letters. In your welcome line do your best to personalize and avoid a generic/archaic introduction (e.g., "To Whom It May Concern," or "Dear Sir or Madam"). This includes using the appropriate title and credentials (e.g., "Dear Dr. Smith" or "Dear Mrs. First Name Last Name, LMHC).

Your cover letter will not have formal sections/headings like your résumé, and there is generally a wider range of accepted approaches in what and how content is presented. The following are common suggestions to help get you started. Your first paragraph should include a brief introduction of yourself (it is okay to include your name even if provided in the header) and reference the job position you are interested in. Your second paragraph (or continued from your first paragraph) should include the name of the college/university and program you are matriculated in (or recently graduated from), including any concentrations and anticipated graduation date. Although it may be obvious based on your application, it does not hurt to state that you are pre-licensure and looking to get more experience and work toward licensure.

Your next paragraph can include your recent counseling experience, including your practicum/internship. This is where you can highlight relevant accomplishments and experiences that connect you to the job position and agency. You can also include other work or research experience that highlight applicable skills in relation to the job position. Try not to let your fear of bragging get in the way. Sometimes early-career counselors (or perhaps it is a personality trait) feel like highlighting accomplishments and counseling skills is being too full of oneself. Being humble is a good personal trait to have. However, the people reviewing your application want to see what makes you stand out from other applicants. If you are too reserved, you will not come off as unique, even though you are. Do your best to find a comfortable balance between being modest and providing a full picture of how you can benefit the agency.

The final paragraph can include a brief summary of your personal skills and traits. In other words, who you are as a person, not just as a counselor. Do your best to avoid using vague, fluffy statements like "team player" or "people person." Instead, describe what these qualities look like in you. Keep in mind that it is common for some individuals while writing this section to talk about how the agency is great and will benefit them. A few brief comments like this are okay, but it is most important to highlight what you can provide the agency (they already know what they can give you!). If it helps, remember to think of what John F. Kennedy might say: "Ask not what your agency can do for you, ask what you can do for your agency." If you focus too much on what the agency can give you, it can be a turnoff to those reviewing your application. Finally, conclude with a brief statement thanking them for their time to review your application and stating that you look forward to hearing back from them. You can also include the best way they can reach you, if this is not provided in your résumé. Of course, also include your signature at the end.

Activity 5.3: Résumé and Cover Letter Draft

If you have not done so already, it is time to develop a draft of your résumé and cover letter. If it helps, you can use Box 5.1 (résumé example) and Box 5.2 (cover letter example) as templates. Although you have your own style, do your best to follow the above basic formatting and key components suggestions specific to clinical mental health job positions. If it helps provide context, consider one of the job positions from your job search when making your drafts. This can increase motivation, knowing that your drafts will serve an actual purpose in finding a job. Remember to have at least a couple individuals review your résumé and cover letter drafts for spelling/grammar and overall presentation.

Box 5.1 ▪ Résumé Example

Elizabeth Erd
Worcester, MA
lizerd@university.edu
123-456-7890 (work)

EDUCATION

Master of Arts, Clinical-Counseling Psychology Anticipated May 2022
Concentration: Child and Family Interventions
Assumption University, Worcester, MA
GPA: 3.8
Bachelor of Arts, Psychology May 2020
Fitchburg State University, Fitchburg, MA
GPA: 3.6, Magna Cum Laude

PROFESSIONAL AFFILIATIONS

American Mental Health Counselors Association 2018 to Present
Psi Chi, National Honor Society, Fitchburg State University 2017 to Present

COUNSELING EXPERIENCE

John Smith Youth & Family Services, Worcester, MA May 2021 to Present
Practicum and Intern Counselor
Supervisor: John Smith, LMHC

- Conducted weekly individual, family and group therapy sessions with children, adolescents, and families diagnosed with a variety of disorders including adjustment disorders, ADHD, oppositional defiant disorder, major depressive disorder, bipolar disorder, anxiety disorders, and posttraumatic stress disorder
- Provided CBT and evidence-based family interventions for youth and their families
- Received training in basic DBT interventions
- Maintained a case load of approximately 10–12 weekly clients
- Diagnosed and developed and wrote treatment plans, process notes, and diagnostic summaries
- Co-facilitated two anger management groups for middle school males and high school students; conduct prescreening intake interviews to assess appropriateness for group membership
- Assisted with evaluating adolescent females involved with juvenile, including CHINS and care and protection
- Participated in case consultations and crisis interventions
- Organized and participated in fundraisers for the agency including establishing relationships with local vendors and ensuring their continued support, obtaining donated prizes, registration and ticket sales, and event marketing

Box 5.1 ■ Continued

Jane Smith Family Services Gardner, Gardner, MA October 2019 to May 2021
In-Home Family Counselor
Supervisor: Jane Smith, LICSW
- Taught independent living and self-help skills to disadvantaged individuals and families
- Helped clients in developing social skills through practical experiences
- Aided family members in practicing conflict resolution skills
- Completed intake assessments for clients and recommended appropriate treatment plans and maintained accurate case notes documenting client progress

WORK EXPERIENCE

Behavior Intervention Camp, Amherst, MA May 2018 to August 2018
Camp Counselor
- Planned and facilitated groups for adolescents with behavior difficulties
- Enforced delinquency prevention policies and procedures
- Created educational materials and trained camp volunteers

VOLUNTEER EXPERIENCE

Domestic Violence Resource Center, Fitchburg, MA January 2018 to May 2018
Volunteer Advocate
- Served as a liaison between law enforcement officials and distressed family members
- Offered appropriate resources and referrals to victims and families
- Completed specialized trainings for serving victims, including ethical and legal considerations

Peer Educator and Tutor September 2017 to December 2017
Fitchburg Community Education Center, Fitchburg, MA
- Developed course curriculums and taught bimonthly lessons
- Tutored at-risk high school students in psychology and communication courses
- Created learning manuals and assisted students in developing study skills

RESEARCH EXPERIENCE

Assumption University, Psychology Department, Worcester, MA
May 2020 to August 2021

Psychology Research Assistant to Dr. Super Duper
- Participated in two research studies looking at the relationship with empathy and self-control and the attachment between children and their primary caregiver
- Formulated procedures for running the experiments and the schedule for events of the project
- Reported, analyzed, and input the relevant data for both studies
- Presented findings to professors, peers, and administrators in various settings
- Ran the experiments independently and trained peers in proper procedures and format for future experiments
- Learned the IRB procedure for approval with special attention paid to ethical considerations and many other aspects of the research process

OTHER RELEVANT SKILLS
- Microsoft Office Suite 97, 2000, XP (Microsoft Word; PowerPoint; Excel; Publisher)
- Standard First Aid (2016 to Present, American Red Cross, Worcester, MA)
- Nonviolent Crisis Prevention Certified
- SPSS Software

Box 5.2 ■ Cover Letter Example

Elizabeth Erd
Worcester, MA
lizerd@university.edu
123-456-7890 (work)

March 22, 2022

Dr. Milo Foster, Director, Mental Health Unit
City State Correctional Facility
12 Main Street
Townsville, MA 01234

Dear Dr. Foster,

I had the opportunity to meet Jane Doe, one of your licensed mental health counselors, at a professional meeting last fall. I will be graduating with a Master of Arts degree in Clinical-Counseling Psychology from

Box 5.2 ■ Continued

Assumption University in May 2022. I am applying for a recent job posting on your website titled "correctional mental health counselor." I am very interested in working with female populations within a correctional setting. Through my graduate-level internship at John Smith Youth and Family Services, I have gained experience evaluating and counseling adolescent females involved in the juvenile justice system. After Jane and I talked about her work at City State Correctional Facility, my interest in pursuing a mental health counseling career in the correctional system was further reinforced.

Through my academic training and practical experience, I believe I have a solid initial foundation in counseling techniques and approaches that would assist the women at City State. I have an interest in trauma work and understand that much of the work with this population is related to abuse, trauma, and PTSD. I am trained in cognitive-behavioral therapy through my graduate program and have had exposure to dialectical behavior therapy through my recent internship. There, I assisted in evaluating adolescent females involved with the Juvenile Court on Delinquency, CHINS, care and protection-related matters, and participated in case consultations, crisis intervention, treatment planning, and resource referrals. My experience throughout this internship was challenging but rewarding. It is my goal to continue to work with individuals who need support as they rebound from past trauma, and learn life skills and coping strategies that will help them to live healthier lives when they re-enter society.

I am confident that my education and experience will allow me to serve as a well-qualified provider for your agency. I am a conscientious individual who is open to learn and gets along well with people from diverse backgrounds. Even as a recent graduate I believe that I can contribute to your mission of "providing new opportunities to reintegrate," including my developing counseling skills of using evidence-based practice integrated with genuine empathy. The women at City State deserve to receive quality mental health treatment while they are inmates that will assist with their overall rehabilitation.

I would welcome the opportunity to discuss my qualifications with you in person. I can be reached at 123-456-7890 or by email at lizerd@university.edu. Thank you for your time and consideration. I look forward to hearing from you.

Sincerely,

_____

Elizabeth Erd

Reflection Questions 5.5: Résumé and Cover Letter Draft Review

- Was creating your résumé and cover letter an enjoyable or unpleasant process? Explain what you were thinking and feeling while creating both documents.
- Were there any particular sections of the résumé or cover letter that were more challenging than others (e.g., from formatting to key components suggestions)? Explain.
- What parts of your résumé and/or cover letter could use some improvement (e.g., experience, description of duties)?
- Are you confident in your résumé and cover letter being an accurate representation of your professional experience and overall image? Explain. How do you think potential employers will respond to these documents?
- What are your thoughts about continuously updating your résumé (e.g., every 3–4 months)?

MANAGING YOUR ONLINE REPUTATION

So, you have begun your job search via the Internet and/or social networking and made your résumé and at least one cover letter. You are now ready to submit your first application and wait for your first interview. Well, not so fast. You may not know this, but you already have a résumé available for potential employers, and it is online! Before you hit the submit button for the first time it is wise to review your online reputation. There could be a few things on there that might put you in a compromising position. At best, you might have just a few silly pictures of you and your friends. At worst, you might have some very strong statements and/or compromising pictures. Some of this content may have been willingly posted by yourself. Other content may have been posted by others unknown to you. Be most concerned about any content that can be perceived negatively by others. In short, you do not want to look like a buffoon or a bigot (or both). (If you really do think you are a buffoon or a bigot, please refrain from being a mental health counselor.)

The reality is that "back in the day" prospective employees did not have to worry about the Internet because it did not exist. Even during the early years of the Internet there was not much for social media and "posting" of content. You could omit anything you did not want your potential employer to see on your résumé and cover letter. There were no little dirty secrets out there or anything embarrassing or greatly regrettable available for the public eye. You were what they saw on paper (yes, literally paper) until you received an interview. The good ole days... Now you are being interviewed online before interviewing face-to-face. The good news is that there are things you can do to improve your online reputation and minimize the chance for future damaging content.

Your Online Interview

Each year it has become increasingly common for potential employers to use the Internet to screen candidates before offering an interview (Career-Builder, 2018). In some ways, your online presence is like a preinterview; or you can call it an online interview. This means that if a potential mental health agency likes your résumé and cover letter, they will most likely first interview you online and then determine if they want to interview you face-to-face. With a face-to-face interview you at least know it is coming in advance and can prepare. An online interview can happen at any time and you cannot prepare unless you have already "washed" your online presence in advance.

If you are still not convinced, consider the following. The Harris Poll completed a survey on behalf of CareerBuilder using 1,012 hiring and human resource managers between April 4 and May 1, 2018 (CareerBuilder, 2018). Seventy percent of employers reported that they utilize social media

Table 5.3   Online Reputation Reasons for Employers Not Hiring Job Candidates

CareerBuilder (Harris Poll)	Jobvite (Recruiter Nation Report)
• Provocative or inappropriate photographs, videos, or information (40%) • Information about self—drinking or using drugs (36%) • Discriminatory comments related to race, gender, or religion (31%) • Linked to criminal behavior (30%) • Lied about qualifications (27%) • Poor communication skills (27%) • Negative comments about previous employer or fellow employee (25%) • Unprofessional screen name (22%) • Shared confidential information from previous employers (20%) • Lied about an absence (16%) • Posted too frequently (12%)	• Marijuana use in the last year (61%) • Political rants (51%) • Spelling/grammar errors (48%) • Alcohol consumption (35%) • Showing off wealth/big purchases (19%) • Showing too much skin (16%) • Limited social presence (12%) • Posting many selfies (7%)

to screen candidates prior to hiring. This was up from 11% in 2006. In addition, 66% use online search engines (e.g., Google, Yahoo!, and Bing) to screen candidates as well. Even though these statistics are based on employers across all fields, it is prudent to consider that mental health agencies are engaged in similar screening processes as well. It should be clear that your online presence cannot be ignored.

Looking at your online presence is one thing, but how much it impacts the hiring process is more relevant. Overall, the Harris Poll found that 54% of employers discovered content on social media that resulted in them not hiring a candidate for an open position (CareerBuilder, 2018). The real learning comes from knowing what these employers see that turns them off from hiring job candidates. Table 5.3 provides the major reasons for employers not hiring candidates based on the Harris Poll. It also includes the major reasons that give job recruiters a negative impression of candidates according to Jobvite's "2017 Recruiter Nation Report" (Jobvite, 2017).

Based on the findings of these two surveys, it is best to not do/post the following online: use or be associated with drugs and alcohol, especially in an immature manner; making comments about race, gender, religion, or strong political views/rants; provocative or inappropriate photos or videos, usually too much skin, sexual or violent in nature; poor spelling/grammar and/or poor communication skills (do not use "texting language"); negative comments about previous/current employer or fellow employee (or client!); dishonesty about qualifications; associated with criminal behavior; unprofessional screen name (including email address); showing off wealth; limited social presence or too much of a social presence (i.e., too many posts). Hopefully, you did not check off too many boxes while reading these turnoffs. With that said, even if one of these reasons relates to you, do your best to take care of it as soon as possible (discussed next). If you think that you have something online that was not in the list, but you are not sure if it is appropriate, then it probably is not. Make it go away. The last thing you want to happen is to not get an interview for a job that you know you are well qualified for because of something stupid posted on the Internet. Worst of all, if you do not receive an interview offer, you might not even know it was because of what was found online (those reviewing your application do not have to tell you why). Of course, there are some things from your past that you might not have much control over, like a criminal record. This is really a separate topic, but at the very least it is usually best to be upfront about it in the beginning. Finally, you may have noticed that some employers/recruiters had concerns about having too much or too little of a social presence—you cannot win! Do not worry much about this when applying for mental health counselor jobs. As long as your online content is appropriate you will be fine. If you do not have much of an online presence, or even if you do, it is a good idea to at least have a LinkedIn account (discussed soon).

Your online presence does not have to have only a negative effect on your job search. The other side of the coin is also possible: an employer could offer you an interview/job because of something they liked on your social media or through an online search. According to the Harris Poll, 44% of employers found content on a social media that positively influenced their decision to hire a candidate (CareerBuilder, 2018). The reasons for hiring the candidate included professional qualifications supported (37%), creativity (34%), good professional image (33%), and great communication skills (28%). Relatedly, job recruiters reported that examples of work (65%), engagement in volunteering, mentoring, or nonprofits (63%), and mutual connections (35%) were top factors to offer a candidate an interview (Jobvite, 2017). Essentially, being able to express yourself well online, appropriately communicate well with other people, and help others in need puts you in an attractive position for potential employers. Mental health counseling agencies are especially interested in making sure their potential employees have good interpersonal skills, as this is very important for working with both colleagues (i.e., "Is this someone I want to work with?") and clients (e.g., "Is this someone who can establish rapport with clients and help them?").

An interesting footnote to keep in mind is that once you are hired, you still need to stay vigilant with your online content. The Harris Poll reports that 48% of employers use social media sites to research their current employees (CareerBuilder, 2018). Of these employers, 34% found concerning content online that resulted in either reprimanding or firing an employee. Although there are many reasons that can cause concern from your employer, posting negative comments about your agency, colleagues, or clients will most likely result in some negative attention. Also, making racist, bigoted, or political rants also will have a negative outcome. The moral of this data is, do not let your guard down once hired. Furthermore, you never know when you might be looking for a new job or a recruiter is looking for you. In other words, even when employed you can still be a potential job applicant.

Reflection Questions 5.6: Your Online Interview Thoughts

- What are your thoughts about potential employers searching your social media and the Internet to find additional information about you? Is this surprising to you or expected?

- Are the many reasons for employers/recruiters not hiring candidates concerning to you? Are they being "fair" in their decision process? Does fairness matter?
- Your online content can also have a positive influence on employers/recruiters. What information about you is currently readily available that may leave a positive impression?

Manage Your Online Reputation like a Car Wash: Clean, Protect, and Polish

You might be thinking that it is best to get rid of all your online presence as much as possible. You also probably know that this is not realistic. Some information, for better or worse, will always be available for others to see. However, there is some information that you can truly delete or at least modify. You can also implement strategies to help minimize any potential future mishaps. As noted earlier, many potential employers prefer that you have an online presence. The Harris Poll found that 47% of employers are less likely to contact a candidate for an interview if that candidate cannot be found online (CareerBuilder, 2018). Of these employers, 20% expect candidates to have an online presence and 28% prefer to obtain additional information (i.e., online interview) before scheduling an interview with the candidate. Thus, instead of avoiding the Internet, embrace it and do your best with what you have. Try to look at maintaining your online presence like going to a car wash. You first want to clean as much filth off the car as possible (knowing that some filth and scratches may still remain). Next, you want to use protective solutions to help minimize further filth buildup and future scratches. Finally, you do your best to polish your car to make it look as shiny as possible. A clean and shiny car is more attractive than a filthy and scratched-up car!

Clean

Now is as good a time as any to start cleaning your online reputation. Remember, you are supposed to be a professional, and how you present yourself to others is important. The first thing to do is go through all your social media–related accounts (e.g., Instagram, Facebook, LinkedIn [discussed later], Myspace [just kidding!], Pinterest, Twitter, YouTube) and Google yourself. When you Google yourself, use other related key words (e.g., your hometown, high school, university), especially if you have a common name. This also includes variations of your name and common misspellings. You might be surprised by what you find. Remove everything (i.e., comments/tweets, pictures, videos, "un-like," de-tag) that was identified in Table 5.3 and anything else that makes you pause for a moment.

Go through your profile for each of these websites and not only remove any inappropriate information, but also rewrite any sections that may need to be enhanced with more appropriate content while also highlighting your own personality and strengths. If possible, without coming off as contrived, showcase yourself in a manner that exemplifies someone that is a professional mental health counselor (e.g., empathic, caring, thoughtful, approachable, nonjudgmental).

You might find that there is some information that is either very difficult or impossible to remove. Before giving up, consider doing an internet search on how to remove content from specific websites; perhaps you are missing or not understanding some of the features. If it is possible, somebody has probably already done it and posted instructions. Keep in mind, this cleaning only relates to websites that you have at least some control over. There is not much you can do about content posted by other parties (e.g., city newspaper that has a short article about your recent DUI). These may be things you have to live with. There are some organizations that will try to remove such content. Try doing an internet search like "manage my online reputation" or something similar. However, keep in mind these services can be very expensive.

Protect

Once you have cleaned up your online presence, ensure that you minimize the chances of any unwanted information appearing in the future. The short response is to simply stop posting, commenting, liking, and tagging inappropriate content. This can be challenging for some people. A good suggestion is that before you post something when emotionally aroused, try to wait at least a few hours to a day and/or type/write it out. Many times, when people post something that might be considered inappropriate, it is when they are experiencing an extreme emotional state: very happy, very sad, very mad, or too much to drink or smoke. (As you probably know by now, you cannot blame alcohol or Ambien for a racist or political rant!) Thus, it is best to revisit your desire to post after you have calmed down (or sobered up). Also, if you do make a mistake and are aware of it, you can always remove that post before it causes too much damage, assuming it is before someone takes a screenshot.

There are some things you might not have control over, such as your friends or family posting content about you. What you can do is respectfully request that they ask your permission before posting anything about you online. Hopefully they can respect your request; but if it helps, you can explain that it is for your own benefit in establishing yourself as a mental health counselor professional who is looking to obtain and maintain a job. If it is a social media website, you do have control over your privacy settings (e.g., who can see your account, permission to tag you, permission to share post/tweet, ability to post on your page). You may even want to disable location services when attending social events to provide some additional privacy (or permanently disable location services). How much control you truly have depends on the social media account. At the very least, take advantage of all the privacy options you reasonably can.

Polish

Your cleaning and protecting should not be a one-shot event. Early in your career, review the content and privacy settings of your social media accounts and do an online search of yourself every 1–3 months. Take this time to also review your profiles and provide any necessary revisions and updates with new information. Having an outdated profile could be a turnoff to potential employers. Just like your résumé, your online presence is a continuous working document. Finally, be aware that some social media accounts are known to modify their privacy settings unbeknownst to you. Make sure the privacy settings are still the way you want them to be and see if there are additional features/settings you can take advantage of. If you have a system in place to "keep tabs" on the process, it is not too overwhelming; it can actually be enjoyable. When you let things go, it becomes a stressful and unpleasant task.

If you do not already have a LinkedIn account, get one. More than 766 million people have a LinkedIn profile—over 171 million of them in the U.S. (Omnicore, 2021). It is often the first site potential employers visit if they are curious about you. This is a good thing because LinkedIn is a professional ("business-like") account that allows you to show your education, work/volunteer experiences, and other skills. Although there is an option to post information, it is professional in nature. This is not a site where you show your personal life. A LinkedIn profile is generally a safe place for employers to view all your content. You can even post a personal photo here—it is expected! Although it is not too common in the mental health field, this is also where agency headhunters can find you (i.e., "passive-job-seekers"). Agencies may be looking for you when you are not looking for them. Therefore, it is wise to complete as many sections as you can for your LinkedIn profile. You can even attach your résumé, presentations or publications, and links to your personal website or blog. In this case, your LinkedIn profile can only help you. Finally, as you get more connections on LinkedIn, the more your professional social network expands. These "links" may someday become helpful for networking future job positions. Additionally, LinkedIn has forums (i.e., groups) that are organized by content of interest. These groups can keep you in touch with other mental health counselors with similar professional interests/specialties. Again, another great opportunity to network.

Activity 5.4: Managing Your Online Reputation: Give It a Car Wash

Simply take the time to follow the steps to manage your online reputation like a car wash: clean, protect, and polish. Get rid of as much inappropriate content as possible, while also modifying your social media settings to minimize association with inappropriate content. If you do not already have a LinkedIn account, strongly consider this option and review the website and other people's accounts. If you do have a LinkedIn account, take the time to review it like your social media accounts. Not only clean it up, but also polish it by providing a full, detailed, and accurate professional profile. Also put in place a plan to review your online reputation at least every 1–3 months.

Reflection Questions 5.7: Managing Your Online Reputation Review

- Was there any content that you decided to remove? What was it? Was it clearly inappropriate or done out of an abundance of caution?
- Did you notice any content associated with you but not fully under your control (e.g., friend posting picture on social media website)? Were you able to get the content removed? What was this process like?
- What are your thoughts about having a LinkedIn account? If you have a LinkedIn account, discuss how you have found it beneficial to your job search or networking.
- How confident are you that you will be able to maintain appropriate online content over time? If not confident, what can you do?

INTERVIEWING

After you submit your résumé and cover letter, your only real option is to wait. It may take a few weeks to hear back from an agency. Keep in mind that at this point in the hiring process most employers will not contact you to let you know that you did not make it to the interview stage. In some cases you could contact the agency on the status of your application. They will most likely tell you that you will hear back from them later if they are interested. If they tell you that the position has already been filled, then you have your answer; you will not be having an interview. Also, they most likely will not tell you why you were not invited for any interview. Potential employers will only sometimes give feedback after the interview stage (even then, do not expect much). If you applied to a position through networking with someone privy to the hiring process, you might be able to receive some feedback.

Remember, all mental health agencies want to interview and hire potential candidates with the least amount of risk, including their time and resources. At this stage of the application process, it really is more about elimination than hiring. This is why you want to make sure your résumé, cover letter, and online reputation are as strong as possible. You want to get your foot inside the door to make your next impression through interviewing. Once you are invited for an interview, the process becomes more about hiring than elimination. You now know that they at least like you on paper. Now you have to present yourself in person and demonstrate you are someone worth hiring.

You might have some strong thoughts and emotions about the prospect of being invited to an interview, either positive or negative. Although you have probably interviewed for other positions in the past, this interview will most likely feel different, as it is your first potential employment as a mental health counselor. You not only have to support the content of your résumé and cover letter during the interview, you will also be asked questions to demonstrate your interpersonal skills and problem-solving skills. You might even be asked to role-play or complete a writing assignment. An interview at this stage of your career is serious. But that does not mean it should be stressful and unpleasant. It might even be fun!

You may find it helpful to organize your thinking and preparation by viewing interviewing as having three main stages: before, during, and after. The before part is how you respond when contacted by an agency for an interview and what you do to prepare for the interview. During the interview includes how you present yourself, communicate, and answer and ask questions. What you do after the interview focuses on processing the interview experience, maintaining communication, and responding to job offers and rejections.

Before Your Interview: Research and Practice

An old cliché line is that "interviewing for a job is a lot like dating." The reason for this line being cliché is because it is true. You are hoping the agency likes you and, if the interview goes well, the agency hopes you like them. Of course, this means both of you are trying to present yourselves in the best way possible (i.e., courting). At this point, the courting has largely been one-sided (i.e., you trying to impress the agency) and will most likely remain this way until at least the interview stage. With that said, not only remember to keep presenting your best self, but also know that you have your options and do not have to settle. This means you can start observing in more detail your likes/dislikes (or strengths/weaknesses) of any agencies you may interview with. Once offered an interview, it is wise to do some further research on the agency while also practicing for your first date. Be sure to prepare for all interviews to give yourself the best chance of being hired.

Look at it this way, your application with résumé and cover latter was like asking the agency for a first date—you initiated the potential relationship. When the agency contacts you for an interview, they are agreeing to a first date, ideally with not too much trepidation. This first contact, even if a simple email or voicemail, should be treated seriously. You are both now courting in a more personal nature. This means, respond to the interview offer in a professional manner. First, if an email or voice message is left for you, respond within 24–48 hours (or sooner). Be respectful in your response and be as flexible as possible in scheduling your interview. Even though your correspondence may be brief, the agency is already "sizing you up." For example, are you pleasant to talk to and flexible? Furthermore, do you sound confident or desperate (or overly anxious, insecure) during your conversation? Ideally, if you are returning a call, take a look at your calendar over the next 2–3 weeks and take note of the days/times you will be available. Additionally, keep in mind, if you do not screen your phone calls, you might immediately talk to someone from the agency rather than an initial voicemail. If this is a possibility with your phone habits, keep a written log of each agency you have applied to with a few notes on hand (see Table 5.2 reviewed earlier) in order to avoid being caught off guard. To be safe, this really is a good time to screen your calls. (Remember to make sure your voicemail message is clear and appropriate!)

After an agency contacts you to schedule an interview, begin taking notes (literally and figuratively) including initial impressions, strengths/weaknesses, and questions. Now is the time to review your initial notes and do a more thorough review of each agency that has offered you an interview. Review the agency website and peruse each page. Take a look at the description for each department and/or services provided. Review any staff/administrative profiles. There may also be additional information such as client testimonials, social media postings of recent work done in the community, trainings, and research. Be sure to review the agency's mission statement and anything else that speaks to their values (e.g., "about us").

Websites like Glassdoor can also be helpful in understanding agency culture through employee comments and client comments. This information does have value, especially if you notice patterns from multiple posters. However, keep in mind that this information may not be fully accurate or objective. There may be sampling bias of those that post. Typically, individuals who are not happy with their employment or services received are more likely to post negative comments/reviews. A general search of the Internet may also yield additional information, such as work done in the community and political activism/social justice for the profession and clients served. Finally, be sure to take advantage of any information your contacts (i.e., networking through colleagues, professors, other individuals in the field) may have about the agency.

All this information can give you a preliminary understanding of the agency's core values, culture, and overall approach to treating their employees and clients. This can also give a sense for potential "fit" within the agency, including both your own personal values and approach to counseling. Review the specific job position you applied for and the résumé and cover letter you provided to the agency. You want to highlight how your skills match the job you are applying for. While doing this, try to consider how you can contribute to the agency's mission and goals, including client care. Integrating this information into your interview can give a positive impression. Consider preparing a list of agency-specific and general questions to ask during your interview (discussed later). All of this shows you took initiative and did your homework.

Activity 5.5: Interview Research

Table 5.4 is a simple template for you to take notes for each agency interview. Each row provides space to list the name of the job position and a brief description. Next, there are columns to provide more detailed information such as your relevant skills related to the position and your initial impressions of the agency, including agency strengths and weaknesses. You can also record any agency-specific questions you may want to ask during the interview. The final column can be used after the interview to follow up on your initial thoughts and impressions. There are some similarities here to Table 5.2. You can carry over some of the information from Table 5.2 to this template and expand upon your thoughts, impressions, and questions now that you know you will be interviewing for specific agencies. This template will also make it easier to compare other agencies if you have multiple interviews and, possibly, multiple offers.

Table 5.4   Interview Research and Reflection Template

| | Relevant Skills | Agency | | | | Post-Interview Thoughts & Impressions |
		Initial Impressions	Strengths	Weaknesses	Specific Questions	
1. Job Title _____ Description _____ _____ _____						
2. Job Title _____ Description _____ _____ _____						
3. Job Title _____ Description _____ _____ _____						

Reflection Questions 5.8: Interview Research Review

- How well do your skills match up for each job position? What skills could give you a competitive advantage relative to other early-career mental health counselors?
- Does anything stick out about your initial impressions for any agency or job position? Do you notice any patterns across agency or job position?
- Based upon your list of strengths and weaknesses, what agency or job position qualities appear to be most and least attractive?
- Is there a theme to the types of questions you would like to ask during the interview? Are your questions more about the agency itself or the job position? What could this possibly mean to what is of most interest to you and how you will approach the interview?

During Your Interview: What You Say and Do (and Not Say and Do)

You were contacted to schedule your interview, and you did your research and maybe practiced (see **Activity 5.6** below). The day of your interview is now here. In other words, this is your first date with your potential agency. As you probably know, fair or not, first impressions go a long way; and there is no second chance to make a first impression. Your first impressions begin the moment you set foot on the agency's property and walk into the building. Thus, it is important to be cognizant of how you present yourself. Obviously, how you communicate to others, verbally and nonverbally, will leave a lasting impression. A key part of communicating during the interview is how you respond to questions and the type of questions you ask. The more you learn about the agency, the more informed you will be in making a decision if given an offer.

How You Present Yourself

Get a good night's sleep. Try to maintain your normal night routine and give yourself the hours of sleep you require to feel refreshed. This means no "all nighter" doing last-minute interview prepping. This should not be necessary if you plan ahead. If you are overtired, you are more likely to behave awkwardly (e.g., trip on your own feet walking upstairs, spill your double espresso coffee, or fart), say something inappropriate (e.g., accidently swear, self-disclose too much, or profess your affections for the receptionist), or simply look like a disaster (e.g., zombie eyes, zipper down, or ramen noodles in your hair). Basically, you will be making a horrible first impression before your formal interview even starts. The date is over before it even begins.

To give yourself a good start to your interview, not only allow for enough hours of sleep, give yourself enough time to get ready without having to rush. Take a shower. Comb/brush your hair (or beard/mustache). Groom other parts that require grooming. If you use makeup, keep it on the light to moderate side. Brush your teeth and use mouthwash (and take some mints, especially if you smoke). Put on deodorant if you are sweaty, especially when anxious. Use eye drops if your eyes tend to stay red for a long period of time after you wake up or if you have allergies. It is best to lay off the perfume/cologne/aftershave. Some people are allergic or just do not like it. Make sure you dress professionally. There are near-infinite opinions on what men and women should wear to an interview. For most mental health agencies, you do not have to dress formally, but it is best to at least follow business-casual. When in doubt, it is always best to dress a little more on the "business" side of the business-casual (i.e., a little more conservatively). In case you are wondering, this means no T-shirts, jeans, sneakers, or flip-flops!

Bring some type of professional purse/bag/briefcase (not the kind with metal locks; that is weird) to carry basic items like a binder with agency information, including questions you want to ask during the interview. Also bring additional paper and a pen/pencil for notes. It is also wise to bring extra copies of your résumé. Potential interviewers may not have your résumé immediately on hand, but it looks good on your part if you have a few extra copies. Also bring a separate list of references to have on hand, if requested. If you are someone who gets dry mouth when talking a lot, it is okay to bring a bottle of water. Some suggest that bringing a beverage is a turnoff, but most professionals in the mental health field understand the importance of water while on the job.

Know the agency's address and plan to arrive at least 15 minutes early. These days with Google Maps and GPS systems, there is no reason to be late to an interview unless there is some serious unexpected traffic or accident. If you are only a few minutes early, there is nothing wrong with entering the agency's building and letting the receptionist know you have arrived for an interview. (If you know in advance, let the receptionist know who you will be interviewing with.) If you arrive too early (15 or more minutes), it is okay to wait a little longer in your car. If you are very early (30 or more minutes), it might be best to drive around and find another place (e.g., coffee shop) to take up some time; it might be a bit creepy sitting in the parking lot for more than 30 minutes.

Remember that you are interviewing with the whole agency. This begins with the receptionist and any other employee you may interact with. All these individuals are potential colleagues. It is naive to think that being curt with the receptionist will not get back to those involved in the hiring process.

In fact, how you treat others who are not part of your formal interview can go a long way because it is perceived to be a better representation of your personality and how you interact with others than your formal interview. Simply be polite and respectful, including good eye contact and smiling.

Of course, you do not have to be sleep deprived to behave or communicate in an awkward or inappropriate manner. Table 5.5 provides a list of examples that are reported to be "deal-breakers" or turnoffs by recruiters and employers (Jobvite, 2017). Some of these turnoffs may seem obvious, while others appear to be superficial and not fair. You are probably correct. However, this is simply human nature. Fair or not, first impressions can go a long way. Just like dating, interviewers tend to follow the principle of microcosm reflects macrocosm. This is the belief that what you do in a small setting (i.e., interviewee) reveals what you would do in a larger setting (i.e., employee). Finally, note that many of these "turnoffs" are not necessarily major blunders. Sometimes we focus so much on the "big things" we forget how some of the smaller things, especially if they accumulate, can cause the most harm. It is death by a thousand cuts instead of a single thrust through the chest.

Table 5.5 Interview "Deal-Breakers"

Jobvite (Recruiter Nation Report)	Employer Reported
• Rude to receptionist or other support staff (86%) • Checking phone (71%) • Showing up late (58%) • Bad hygiene (52%) • Interrupting the interviewer (39%) • Bringing food (38%) • Too casual dress (24%) • Bringing a beverage (14%) • Bad handshake (6%) • Too much makeup (5%) • Poor fashion (4%) • Not enough makeup (1%)	• Expressing racist/sexist/bigoted attitudes • Appearing intoxicated • Sexual harassment/flirting • Crying • Short interview (less than 10 minutes) • Bringing a child • Not knowing agency interviewing for • Dishonesty • Poor/awkward interpersonal skills • Minimal to no expression of enthusiasm • Ask minimal to no questions • Nervous mannerisms (e.g., avoiding eye contact, constant hand/body fidgeting, playing with hair) • Extreme criticalness toward previous colleagues or employer • Low self-confidence (e.g., self-critical comments, downplay achievements or abilities) • Arrogance • Smoking (includes vaping)

Reflection Questions 5.9: How You Present Yourself Review

- What deal-breakers are the least surprising?
- Are there any deal breakers you find surprising? Explain.
- Are there any deal-breakers that you may be prone to do? What can you do to minimize the chances of engaging in those deal-breakers?
- Do you have any other concerns not addressed about how you may present yourself to those who are interviewing you? Explain.

How You Communicate

Do your best to approach your interview in a way that conveys you are both a person who is pleasant to work with and has good counseling skills. Broadly speaking, this means establishing good rapport with those interviewing you. When the interview is over, you want to be memorable in a positive way and provide a sense of comfort that you are someone they can work with while knowing you will provide quality care to their clients. There is no one way to approach interviewing for a job position in the mental health field. Your own personality and style will naturally influence the impressions you make. However, there are some approaches to communication to consider to minimize the chances for any social/interpersonal blunders. Communication is especially important in the mental health field, considering you are applying for a job that requires counseling clients!

A good start to approaching your interview is to be aware of the Mehrabian Model (Mehrabian & Ferris, 1967; Mehrabian & Wiener, 1967). Mehrabian's study of nonverbal communication found that words account for only 7% of communication. This means the remaining 93% is nonverbal communication. More specifically, voice/tone is 38% and body language is 55%. (Note: there are some valid criticisms of Mehrabian's studies, including context and methodology. Studying verbal and nonverbal communication is a very complex task. With that said, without getting hung up on the specific percentages, focus on the general trend: most of communication is nonverbal, including voice/tone and body language.) The purpose of highlighting nonverbal communication is because it often gets overlooked, even with counselors. It is easy to get hung up on what to say and what not to say. This is still important. Inappropriate or odd comments can end an initially positive interview very quickly. However, inappropriate or odd nonverbal communication can greatly negatively influence the outcome of an interview. The magnitude of the negative impact is often overlooked because of its sometimes subtle or ambiguous nature. Think about it. Have you ever had a conversation with someone who "said all the right things" but you walked away with a funny/odd/uncomfortable feeling? This probably had to do with the nonverbal communication you observed.

There are a few things you can do to monitor your voice/tone. First, simply be aware of the volume of your voice. Some individuals are naturally loud or only when anxiously excited. This can be especially off-putting if in a small room. Others are naturally quiet or only when anxiously timid. If you are not sure about your volume, try to observe those interviewing you. Do they have the look of someone who wants to turn down a loud radio or are they almost squinting to hear what you are saying? You can also do your best to match the volume of those interviewing you. If you notice that the interviewers are a little on the loud or quiet side, modify your volume accordingly. Second, make sure your words match the context of what you are saying. Insincerity and incongruence can be a major social turnoff. For example, if you sound giddy when discussing trauma work with clients, you will come off as insincere. Or, if you are describing a positive life event but your tone is flat, you will come off as incongruent. Finally, try to avoid other annoying voice/tone mannerisms such as mumbling, dramatic exclamations (e.g., "Oh my God!", "No way!", "That's literally amazing!") or hardly saying anything! In summary, you want those interviewing you to hear you in a comfortable manner and understand what you are saying.

Body language can communicate a lot during an interview. Similar to voice/tone, if what you are saying (and how) does not match your body language, it can also be off-putting. There are a few basic things you can do to monitor your body language. First, smile! (But not too much; that is creepy.) For some, smiling is not natural (work on this) or is significantly reduced when anxious. Even if it hurts your face and you have to think about it, do your best to give an occasional smile, especially when you meet your interviewers. Smiling naturally puts most people at ease and provides a pleasant feeling. Second, provide eye contact. (But do not stare, and remember to blink; not doing so also is creepy.) For some, eye contact is significantly reduced when anxious. Understandably, there can be many cultural differences about when to make eye contact and how long. Try not to worry about this, and simply moderate the frequency and duration of eye contact. Making eye contact helps people feel connected to you. Interviewers are usually turned off only if there is minimal to no eye contact. Overall, appropriate smiling and eye contact communicates sincerity and warmth—very attractive qualities.

There are other elements of body language that can easily be overlooked. Do your best to sit up straight with your chest naturally out. This means no slouching or looking down, which can come off as lazy or arrogant. Occasionally leaning forward is okay, but try to not do this too often or it may be perceived as too eager or aggressive. Do not cross your arms, even if you are cold. Crossing your arms can come off as defensive and unapproachable. Putting your hands behind your back can stifle your body movement and come off as arrogant. Putting your hands in your pocket, especially while sitting, is just odd. Simply keep your arms at your side or on your lap. If you are a natural hand talker, that is okay and can be a positive. Just make sure you are not moving your hands so much that it looks like you are swatting at flies. Do not point. It can be perceived as aggressive. Also make sure your head nodding is moderated. It is good to nod your head at times because it shows agreement and paying attention. Yet, frequent head nodding makes you look silly, like a bobblehead doll. It is okay to verbalize agreement as well. Relatedly, keep in check any possible fidgeting habits you may have: shifting in your chair too much, constantly crossing/uncrossing your legs, tapping/shaking legs, twirling your hair, rubbing your beard/mustache, jingling coins/keys in your pocket, scratching any part of your body, putting your hands up your sleeves, nail biting, picking your nose, and much more! At best these habits will be annoying and you will come off as a nervous Nellie. At worst, these habits will be offensive and you will come off as a creeper. Keeping annoying or odd body movements to a minimum generally conveys maturity and confidence, which are desirable qualities in a mental health setting.

Another important component to communicating during an interview is monitoring how long you talk (or do not talk) and what you talk about. Do your best to observe the "50–50 rule." The more you mix verbally communicating with listening, the better your chances of getting hired. If you talk too much, you might come off as someone who is focused too much on yourself instead of the agency and the clients. If you do not talk enough, you might come off as standoffish and not being fully open and honest about yourself. Similarly, also observe the "20-second to 2-minute rule." When it is your turn to speak, do not speak longer than two minutes or less than twenty seconds. Too much talking may come off as rambling or tangential, and saying too little may come off as being aloof or not having much insight.

When talking about your skills, do your best to provide concrete examples. It can be more effective to "show" your skills instead of "telling." For example, instead of saying you work well with challenging adolescents, follow with an example of specific relationship skills and interventions you used with a client who was initially challenging to establish rapport with. Relatedly, do not focus your conversation too much on what the agency can do for you. Instead, focus more on how you can benefit the agency in a modest manner, both as a colleague and in providing counseling services to clients. You want to come off as confident at your current stage of professional development, but also cognizant that you have a lot to learn (because you really do!). A very attractive quality in the mental health field is counselors who have high self-efficacy in their counseling skills while also being "teachable." In other words, you are open to constructive feedback for growth without being overly defensive.

Reflection Questions 5.10: How You Communicate Review

- Do you have any concerns about your voice/tone? How can you monitor yourself to modulate your voice/tone?
- What are your thoughts about maintaining appropriate smiling and eye contact? Does this come naturally for you or is it something you need to monitor?
- Do you have any nonverbal/fidgeting behaviors that may leave a negative impression during your interview? What are some self-monitoring strategies you can use to minimize these behaviors?
- Do you have any concerns about talking "too much" or "not too much"? What can you do to help balance how much you talk and how much you listen?
- What are some counseling examples that you can share that "show" your skills instead of "telling" them?

How You Answer Questions and Ask Questions

Know the details about the job position and agency. Also know the content of your résumé and cover letter. All this information is fair game. At this point, you should already have done your research and prepared in advance for possible interview questions. You cannot anticipate every question, but preparation will allow for a more natural, confident, and substantive response to most questions. Table 5.6 provides a list of possible agency questions you may be asked during your interview. Notice that the questions are listed in two columns: interview questions common across most professions, and interview questions specific to the clinical mental health counseling profession. Of course, keep in mind that many other questions could be asked of you that are not on this list. Preparing for the questions on this table gives you a solid foundation to answer a variety of questions. Not all your responses have to be perfect; just be sure they are appropriate.

Be sure to always have questions ready to ask the interviewers. You can integrate these questions throughout the interview or ask them at the end, depending on the interview format. Preparing your own questions explicitly demonstrates that you have done your homework and have genuine interest in the agency. Even if you had a very thorough interview and all your questions were naturally answered, ask a few anyway. Not having any questions,

Table 5.6   Possible Agency Interview Questions

Common Questions	Specific to Mental Health Counseling
• Tell me about yourself. • How did you hear about us? • What do you know about this agency? • What do you find attractive about this agency? • Why are you applying for this job? • Tell me about your last job. Why did you leave it? • Give an example of a conflict you had with a colleague and how you handled it. • Where do you see yourself in five years? Ten years? • What are your professional goals? • Give me an example of a time when you set a goal and were able to meet or achieve it. • How would you describe yourself? • What are your major strengths? • What are your greatest weaknesses? • Describe a time you were faced with a stressful situation at work and how you handled it. What else do you do to handle stress? • What are your interests outside of work? • What accomplishments have given you the greatest satisfaction? • Describe how you would be a good team player? • What makes you feel valued at work? • Is there anything else you would like to share about yourself? • Do you have any questions?	• What attracts you to the clinical mental health counseling profession? • Why do you want to work with this population/specialization? • What personal qualities make you (or would make you) a good counselor? • How do you establish therapeutic rapport with your clients? • What would your supervisor say is your strongest counseling skill? • What would your supervisor say is your weakest counseling skill? • What is your theoretical orientation? Explain. • Give a case example using your theoretical orientation (may include formulation, treatment goals, interventions). • What is the most challenging client/case you have ever had? How did you handle it? • What experience do you have in individual/couple/group/family counseling? • What is your experience working with other providers: social workers, nurses, educators, psychologists, psychiatrists? • What is your experience with paperwork/electronic (concurrent) documentation? • What are the most important qualities to you in your counseling supervisor? • What have you found most rewarding so far working in the mental health field? • What do you find most stressful about being a clinical mental health counselor? How do you cope?

especially if asked, can come off as awkward. Just make sure to avoid asking questions that are too obvious and/or have already been clearly answered. Table 5.7 provides a list of possible questions to consider asking during your

Table 5.7   Possible Interview Questions to Ask

Common Questions	Specific to Mental Health Counseling
• What does this job involve beyond the provided job description? • How long has this position been open? • What personality and/or skills do you think are most important for your employees? • How would you describe the culture/climate of this agency? • What is the most stressful aspect of this job? • What do employees find most rewarding about this job? • Is there a lot of turnover? Why do employees leave? • For current employees, how long have they been with the agency? • Do you like to promote within the agency, when possible? • What are the expected days/hours worked? • Am I expected to work overtime? • What benefits are provided? • What is the expected salary? (Okay to ask at end of final interview.) • When should I expect to hear back on your decision? (Okay to ask at end of final interview.)	• What type of evidence-based practices do you use with your populations? • What type of therapy modality will I be providing (e.g., individual, group, family, or couple)? • What can you tell me about the population served (if not clear)? • What counseling skills are vital to effectively treating your client population? • What would be my expected caseload? • What is the background/training of your colleagues (e.g., counselors, social workers, nurses, psychologists, psychiatrists)? • Is pay based on salary or a productivity model? If a productivity model, are my benefits contingent upon it? How does this work? • Will I be on-call (i.e., receive phone calls [possibly for crises] while not working on site; may have to unexpectedly go on site)? • What do you do to support staff self-care and well-being? • Do you provide supervision? Do you have supervisors that are "approved" for my license? Do you have a supervisor with my theoretical orientation? Will supervision be on site? • Do you provide on-site training for specific counseling skills and/or evidence-based interventions? • Do you provide reimbursement for off-site training, including CEUs?

interview. Like the previous table, the questions are listed in two columns: common interview questions to ask in most professions, and interview questions to ask that are specific to the clinical mental health counseling profession. Obviously, you may have your own additional questions to include on your personal list. Whenever possible, try to match your questions to the appropriate person during the interview. Some questions are best left to those in different parts of the hiring process (e.g., human resources, program director, clinical director).

Reflection Questions 5.11: Questions Answered, Questions Asked

- What are your general thoughts and feelings when you are asked questions about yourself and your counseling skills?
- What agency questions are you most concerned/unsure about answering? What can you do to prepare for these questions?
- What questions to ask the agency are most important to you (i.e., the information is vital to your decision to accept or reject a potential offer)?
- What questions are you uncomfortable asking? What are your reasons for feeling this way?

Activity 5.6: Practicing for Your Interview

Some individuals find that they interview naturally, while others need much practice. Perhaps Table 5.2 and Table 5.4 along with the questions in Table 5.6 and Table 5.7 are all the preparation you need. However, many individuals find it helpful to rehearse (e.g., role-play) their interview, especially if anxious. Any type of exposure can help reduce at least some anxiety (just like with your clients!). This can range from simply visualizing your interview to sitting down with a peer or significant other and role-playing an interview from start to finish. Take turns role-playing an interview with at least one of your peers. Take notes for each other, including such observations as voice/tone and nonverbal communication (e.g., fidgety/odd behaviors). You can even video record your role-play to see and hear for yourself what you like and do not like about your interview style. Definitely take the time to practice answering and asking interview questions, especially those you are most concerned about. Process the following questions with your role-play peers based on their feedback and your own observations.

- What are some of your interview strengths? How can you build off these strengths during the interview?
- What were some of your interview weaknesses? Have these weaknesses improved with practice? What other strategies can you use to improve upon these weaknesses?
- What interview skills are you still concerned about? What can you do to continue improving upon these skills?
- If you video recorded your interview, how did this provide additional insight into your strengths and weaknesses?

After Your Interview: Processing, Thanking, Following Up, Offers, and Rejections

Your interview is over, and hopefully it went well. However, you are far from done unless you were told immediately after the interview that you are no longer being considered for the job position (this is rare). Now is the time to process your experience and prepare for future contact.

Process Your Interview Experience

Like any date, courting is a mutual process where not only is the agency determining if you are a good match, but you also should be doing the same with the agency. You may really want the job, but you also want to make sure that you will be happy in the relationship as well. (If you did not enjoy the date, imagine what a long-term relationship would be like!) During the interview, be sure you are making your own assessment about working for the agency. As stated earlier, not only do you want to make a positive impression on those interviewing you, you also want to make sure the agency is a good match for you. Are the job position and duties clear and still attractive to you? Are the interviewers and other employees people you want to work for? It is often easier to note what you liked compared to what you did not like, unless there is something glaring. Pay special attention to the whole context of the interview. Were you interviewed by individuals you will be working with or supervising you? Based on your interactions with the employees (e.g., encouraging and optimistic disposition, made to feel welcomed; or negative expression and tone on their faces, made to feel like an outsider) and environment (e.g., warm and calm atmosphere, well kept; or authoritarian tone of posted signs, disorganized waiting area or office space), did the agency feel positive/hopeful/energetic or depressing/cynical/lethargic? Did they make you feel uncomfortable by asking condescending questions about your education/skills or requesting too much personal information? Any unease or dread you feel may be an early warning sign that something is off. If it helps, review the agency-induced contributing factors to burnout discussed in Table 6.3. You even may have witnessed more explicit inappropriate behavior: last-second canceled interviews (no apology), texting during interviews, racist/sexist jokes, employees/interviewer gossiping/complaining about other employees, flirting with you, much time passes between communication/interview and updates. Some of the more explicit examples of inappropriate behaviors should be disqualifying by themselves. It is not even worth taking a chance to potentially work in such a toxic environment.

Overall, consider the culture and climate of the agency. This should take into consideration your own professional development goals and personal values. No agency will be a perfect match, but some will be much better than others at meeting your professional and personal needs. According to the Recruiter Nation Report, 13% of candidates have turned down a job offer because of agency culture concerns (Jobvite, 2017). For whatever reasons, these individuals did not like the match in values between themselves and the agency. The more your psychological needs, motives, and values are fulfilled, the greater the chances you will be happy, experience job satisfaction, and be invested. Research consistently shows that people's work values are more highly correlated with work satisfaction than with their interests (Rounds, 1990). If you have not done so already, take the time to consider your own values and how they relate to the profession of clinical mental health counseling. If it helps, recall from Chapter 2 that values are generally considered principles or standards of behavior that give our lives meaning. Values are what is important to living a fulfilled life. Formally determining your own personal values is beyond the scope of this text. A suggested source is "The Self-Confidence Workbook" (Markway & Ampel, 2018), which provides a stepwise process to determine your core values. (As you can tell from the title, it is also a great source to work on your self-confidence and self-esteem.) There are also multiple values inventories online. However, be careful in picking one that is well validated. One suggested website is the Life Values Inventory (https://www.lifevaluesinventory. org), authored by Kelly Crace and Duane Brown, both experts in career development.

After the interview, process the experience while reviewing your notes and the answers to your questions. Consider if you noticed any positive or negative patterns. Did your initial experience match up with what was shared to you by other people familiar with the agency, including online reviews? Consider making a list of strengths and weaknesses of the job position and agency. You can also return to Table 5.4, which also includes space to organize your thoughts and feelings after the interview and compare the position to other job positions.

Reflection Questions 5.12: Was the Interview a Good "Date"?

- What did you like most about the interview and agency?
- What did you like least about the interview and agency?
- What are your thoughts about the agency's culture and values? Is it a good match with what you want out of an agency and your values? Explain.
- Did the posted job description match how the job was described during the interview? If no, in what ways are they different?
- Are the salary and benefits acceptable? If no, what could be better?

- What are your overall thoughts and impressions of the agency and job position?
- Do you want to move forward with another date and consider a long-term relationship (i.e., Is this an agency you want to work for?)?

Say "Thank You"

It is best to send a thank-you email later in the day or early the next day. Traditionally, handwritten notes were mailed, but it is now considered socially acceptable to email those that interviewed you. If you do not send a thank-you email, this does not mean you will not be hired. Rather, a well-written thank-you email can leave a small positive impression and helps your interviewers remember you. Your thank-you email should be short in length—typically one paragraph. Mention that you enjoyed the experience and you look forward to hearing back from them. If you can, gently personalize the thank-you by highlighting one or two talking points that connect them to yourself (e.g., enjoyed discussion about serving the homeless in the community, similar conceptualization of client "resistance"). You may or may not receive a reply. Some might give a brief reply about enjoying the interview and contacting you at a future date. Others may say nothing. Do not worry if you do not receive a reply to your thank-you. It is not personal. And do not follow up to see if they received your thank-you; that comes off as desperate.

Following Up

Some interviewees are nervous to follow up after a job interview. This is understandable. You are trying to balance wanting to hear back on a decision without coming off as intrusive. It is okay to follow up; just make sure your timing is appropriate. There is no exact science on when to follow up, but there is a consensus to not follow up before the time frame provided to you. For example, you might be told that you should hear back in a couple of weeks. This should obviously mean to not follow up before two weeks. If you want to be conservative, instead of waiting exactly two weeks for your follow-up wait an extra day or two. Most agencies have no problem with you following up. Of course, be sure your follow-up is respectful and brief. Simply state your name and that you are following up on the status of your application. You will most likely get a response stating that a decision will soon be made or that a decision was made to go with someone else.

Responding to an Offer (or More)

Congratulations! You received a job offer! Assuming that you had time to process your interview experience and you feel like it is a good match, you might want to immediately tell them, "Yes." However, it is often best to thank them and ask for a few days to get back to them. Most agencies do not have a problem with this. They understand that you need time to think it over and might have other options. Your reason for asking for a few days is usually because you want to make sure that this is the right agency for you and/or you have other offers and/or are waiting to hear back from other agencies that might be a better match. If you are fortunate to receive multiple offers, you will need to balance taking the time to review the strengths and weaknesses of each agency and giving your decision to each agency in a timely fashion. The professional thing to do for each offer declined is to contact them within your agreed-upon time frame and respectfully tell them you are no longer interested in the position. It is up to you if you want to tell them that you went with another job offer.

In case you are wondering, there is not much room for salary negotiation for entry-level mental health counselor positions. You may have asked this question toward the end of your final interview. Most agencies have a predetermined salary for non-licensed counselors. You should receive a pay increase once you get licensed and if you are promoted to a supervisor/administrative position. If salary is discussed (which is rare), never state your salary expectations first. It is always best to hear what the agency expects to pay you first. This way, you do not accidentally lowball yourself and you give yourself the opportunity to ask for an increase, especially if the salary seems low compared to that offered by other agencies in your geographic region.

Finally, once you accept an offer, maintain your professionalism up to the first day of work (and onward). It is okay to post on social media that you have accepted a job. With that said, be sure to not post your salary or make any inappropriate comments. Sometimes people are fired from their job before their first day due to inappropriate comments and behaviors. From this point forward, being professional both within the community and on social media should be the norm.

Responding to a Rejection

If you do not get a job offer, that is okay. It is also okay to feel sad or frustrated. However, whether it is by phone or email, be sure to be polite and gracious for the opportunity to interview. You may want to apply to another job at that agency and/or the people you interviewed with probably know individuals that work at other agencies in the community (recall networking). If you feel comfortable and it seems appropriate, you can ask if they have any feedback on how you interviewed. Take note of this information and learn from your experience. You may even be told that there were no major concerns and that they simply went with someone they thought was a better match. This happens. Continue with your job search and interviews. If you are persistent, you will eventually find the right agency for you!

Reflection Questions 5.13: Processing Your Post-Interview Options

- Do you think sending a thank-you email will make a difference in your chances of receiving a job offer? What are some possible benefits?
- What are your thoughts about following up with an agency after the time frame provided. If you are uncomfortable, what are your reasons? What is realistically the worst that can happen?
- What will be the most important agency factors for you to consider when deciding to accept a job offer?
- Will being gracious to a job rejection be challenging for you? What would be your greatest concern? What can you do to ensure that you do not say anything that you might regret later?

REFERENCES

Bolles, R. N. (2018). *What color is your parachute? 2019: A practical manual for job-hunters and career-changers.* Ten Speed Press.

CareerBuilder. (2018). More than half of employers have found content on social media that caused them NOT to hire a candidate, according to recent CareerBuilder survey. Retrieved January 30, 2021 from http://press.careerbuilder.com/2018-08-09-More-Than-Half-of-Employers-Have-Found-Content-on-Social-Media-That-Caused-Them-NOT-to-Hire-a-Candidate-According-to-Recent-CareerBuilder-Survey

Jobvite. (2017). 2017 Recruiter Nation report: Deal-breakers, biases, and best practices: Everything that goes into evaluating the perfect hire. Retrieved January 30, 2021, from https://www.jobvite.com/jobvite-news-and-reports/2017-recruiter-nation-report-evaluating-the-perfect-hire-with-deal-breakers-biases-and-best-practice/Life Values Inventory website: https://www.lifevaluesinventory.org/

Markway, B., & Ampel, C. (2018). *The self-confidence workbook: A guide to overcoming self-doubt and improving self-esteem.* Althea Press.

Mehrabian, A., & Ferris, S. R. (1967). Inference of attitudes from non-verbal communication in two channels. *Journal of Consulting Psychology, 31*, 248–252. https://doi.org/10.1037/h0024648

Mehrabian, A., & Wiener, M. (1967). Decoding of inconsistent communications. *Journal of Personality and Social Psychology, 6*, 109–114. https://doi.org/10.1037/h0024532

Omnicore. (2021). LinkedIn by the numbers: Stats, demographics, and fun facts. Retrieved January 30, 2021, from https://www.omnicoreagency.com/linkedin-statistics/

Rounds, J. B. (1990). The comparative and combined utility of work value and interest data in career counseling with adults. *Journal of Vocational Behavior, 37*, 32–45. https://doi.org/10.1016/0001-8791(90)90005-M

ADDITIONAL RESOURCES

Bernstein. B. (2019). *How to write a killer LinkedIn profile* (14th ed.). Wise Media Group.

Franke, T. (2020). *Interview betterview: A job seeker's essential guide to interview skills*. Roundhouse Recruiting.

Kelley, T. (2017). *Get that job!: The quick and complete guide to a winning interview*. Author.

Ryan, R. (2016). *60 seconds and you're hired!* (Rev ed.). Penguin Books.

6
Self-Care: Preventing Burnout and Enjoying Life

■ ■ ■

Being a mental health counselor and providing effective therapy can instill much fulfillment and many emotional rewards. However, due to the nature of therapy where clients can express intense emotions and share difficult life events, it is not surprising that counselors are prone to experiencing high levels of distress and burnout symptoms. Ironically, the very qualities that contribute to effective counselors (e.g., empathy, caring, compassion) may also contribute to their development of burnout (Lawson et al., 2007). Simply put, one-way caring relationships can be physically and emotionally exhausting if appropriate steps are not taken for self-care.

Although burnout can occur at any stage in your counseling career, research shows that in most cases younger and early-career counselors may be at greater risk than those who are older with many years of experience (Lim et al., 2010; Simionato & Simpson, 2018). This may be because of the lack of exposure to particular traumatic life events that typically come with age and professional experience. In fact, Butler et al. (2017) found in their study of mental health trainees that all participants reported exposure to trauma in their field placements (i.e., practicum, internship) and/or classes, which was associated with burnout and secondary traumatic stress symptoms. Thus, it only makes sense that early-career counselors receive psychoeducation and practice in recognizing symptoms of burnout and enhancing self-care (Kaeding et al., 2017).

Burnout is a concern for not only your own mental health well-being, but also the organizations you work for and the clients you serve. For example, experiencing burnout can result in having off-putting behaviors with your colleagues, reduced efficiency in paperwork/deadlines, and irreparably damaging therapeutic client relationships. In fact, the American Counseling Association (ACA, 2014) and the American Mental Health Counselors Association (AMHCA, 2020) both acknowledge potential ethical concerns that can arise as a result of therapeutic impairment. Others argue that counselor self-care is an ethical necessity and professional responsibility (Norcross & VandenBos, 2018; Wise et al., 2012).

If reading the previous few paragraphs has made you feel a bit despondent, do not despair! You will be happy to know research shows that mental health professionals consistently report high levels of career satisfaction, with very few reporting being very dissatisfied (Lawson, 2007; Norcross & Karpiak, 2012; Walfish et al., 1991). The initial main takeaway here is that most mental health professionals enjoy their profession and derive great purpose and meaning in what they do. With that said, there needs to be recognition that what you do can be stressful and potentially traumatizing. Rather than ignoring this risk or being reactive in nature, it is better to acknowledge it and be proactive in developing self-care.

Before addressing self-care, it important to first define burnout, especially within the context of mental health counselors. Relatedly, the negative impact burnout can have on counselors and their clients is discussed. Additionally, common contributing factors to mental health counselors will be identified. Finally, this chapter will conclude with a discussion of self-awareness/self-monitoring and proactive self-care strategies to prevent burnout and improve overall quality of life.

BURNOUT: WHAT IT LOOKS LIKE IN MENTAL HEALTH COUNSELORS

Before discussing the negative effects of burnout and developing adaptive self-care strategies to avoid this distressing syndrome, it is important to provide a clear operational definition. Although there are many definitions of burnout, researchers and practitioners in the mental health field tend to prefer Maslach and colleagues' (Maslach et al., 2016; Maslach & Goldberg, 1998) multifaceted definition that comprises three dimensions: emotional exhaustion, depersonalization, and reduced personal accomplishment. Emotional exhaustion consists of feelings of being emotionally depleted, overextended, and exhausted in response to the demands of work. Depersonalization (sometimes called compassion fatigue) is a lack of empathy and impersonal response toward those being served. Reduced personal accomplishment consists of low work self-efficacy, including feelings of incompetence and lack of achievement. It does not take much effort to deduce that mental health counselors experiencing burnout are vulnerable to providing substandard care to their clients. Stated differently, counselors have an emotionally taxing job that requires high levels of empathy. If counselors are unable to adequately care for themselves, they will most likely not be able to adequately care for their clients. More specifically, "burned out" counselors are unable to meet the emotional needs of their clients, lack empathy toward their clients' life experiences (to the point where they may be negative or callous), and feel incompetent in their ability to improve the well-being of their clients.

Thousands of studies since the early 1970s have approached measuring work-related burnout using the well-validated Maslach Burnout Inventory (MBI), now in its fourth edition (Maslach et al., 2016). In addition to the original version of the MBI, there are now four additional versions (i.e., medical personnel, educators, general, students). Burnout has been examined across various professions. Of course, one area that has received much attention is the mental health field due to its reputation as a high-stress profession.

Morse et al. (2012) in their review of several studies in the mental health field found that 21–67% of mental health providers reported high levels of burnout. This is not surprising considering the frequency and intensity of the client events mental health providers are exposed to, such as suicidal ideation/attempts, trauma, and hostile interactions (Awa et al., 2010; Sjolie et al., 2015; Zapf et al., 2001). Correspondingly, mental health providers experiencing high levels of burnout are more prone to experience a variety of mental health problems (e.g., depression, anxiety, substance abuse, poor sleep quality) and physical health problems (e.g., cardiovascular disease, neck/back pain, flu-like symptoms, gastroenteritis; Acker, 2010; Maslach et al., 2001; Melamed et al., 2006; Morse et al., 2012; Peterson et al., 2008). This brief summary of the literature may feel a bit daunting. However, keep in mind that not all counselors experience burnout. Furthermore, many of the negative mental and physical health effects occur in those experiencing high levels of burnout over a considerable amount of time (i.e., months or years). Thus, the message here is that recognizing the effects and contributing factors of burnout while also developing healthy self-care strategies can maintain and enhance your well-being while helping you provide quality care to your clients.

BURNOUT IN THE MENTAL HEALTH FIELD: ITS EFFECTS ON MENTAL HEALTH COUNSELORS AND CLIENTS

Burnout can have many negative emotional and physical outcomes. The following highlights the most common symptoms and outcomes experienced by counselors and clients. A key takeaway here is that burnout can affect not only you personally but also your family, friends, colleagues, and clients, the very people you are trying to help.

You, the Mental Health Counselor

There is much literature available on how burnout negatively impacts counselors. Table 6.1 organizes this literature from the perspective of a counselor (Acker, 2010; Bride, 2004; Maslach et al., 2001; Melamed et al., 2006;

Table 6.1   The Impact of Burnout on Mental Health Counselors

Psychological	Behavioral	Physical

• Irritability
• Depression
• Boredom
• Frustration
• Helplessness/
  hopelessness
• Sadness
• Unmotivated/lack
  of purpose
• Apathy
• Unempathetic
• Detachment
• Low therapy
  self-efficacy
• Sense of failure
• Cynicism/
  Disillusionment
• Decreased
  accomplishment
• Exhaustion
• Anxiety
• Poor concentration
• Secondary traumatic
  stress
• Vicarious
  traumatization
	• Substance abuse
	• Overeating
	• Decreased pro-
	  ductivity (billing,
	  paperwork)
	• Procrastination
	• Recklessness
	• Withdrawn
	• Loneliness/isolation
	• Taking frustration
	  out on others (clients,
	  colleagues, family)
	• Calling out from work
	• Coming in late/leaving
	  early from work
	• Interpersonal prob-
	  lems (family, friends,
	  colleagues)
	• Reluctance to check
	  work email/voicemail
	• Lack of focus in
	  sessions
	• Minimal patience with
	  clients
	• Sedentary/passive
	  activities
	• Poor boundaries
	  (work/personal)
		• Poor sleep quality
		• Headaches
		• Muscle aches (e.g.,
		  back/neck)
		• Chronically fatigued
		• Change in appetite
		• Respiratory problems
		• Cardiovascular
		  problems
		• Lowered immunity
		  (often feeling sick)
		• Flu-like symptoms
		• Gastroenteritis

Morse et al., 2012; Peterson et al., 2008; Toppinen-Tanner et al., 2005). More specifically, note that the symptoms are divided up into three domains: psychological, behavioral, and physical. It is acknowledged that not all symptoms neatly fit into each domain and that some symptoms may exacerbate other symptoms (or be part of a larger syndrome) both within and across domains. Furthermore, the line between "warning signs" of burnout and actual symptoms of burnout can be fuzzy. Regardless, based on the plethora of symptoms and varying frequency and intensity, burnout can present in a multitude of ways. There is no one "type" of burnout.

It is important to note here that secondary traumatic stress and vicarious traumatization are both listed under the psychological domain. Secondary trauma occurs when counselors manifest posttraumatic symptoms from constant exposure to clients' traumatic experiences (Butler et al., 2017). Vicarious traumatization is when counselors have a shift in their inner experience (e.g., sense of self, worldview) in relation to the empathic engagement with clients' trauma (Harrison & Westwood, 2009). They are not the same as burnout. However, like other syndromes (e.g., depression, substance abuse), these conditions can develop separately or as part of the consequence of burnout, especially when treating clients with trauma history (Bride, 2004).

Overall, considering all the symptoms in Table 6.1, it should not be surprising that burnout can negatively affect both personal and professional life. If you notice that you are experiencing even just a few of these symptoms, it is probably time to pause and reflect on possible contributing factors, both internal and external. Hopefully, reviewing these symptoms with some personal reflection will put you in a better position to appreciate and be proactive in responding to burnout rather than reactive.

Activity 6.1: Mental Health Counselors and Burnout

Table 6.1 provides an extensive list of the possible impacts of burnout on mental health counselors. Identify at least six symptoms you have experienced, or may be vulnerable to experience, as a mental health counselor. Also note the severity (0–10; minimal to severe) and what domain each symptom falls under (i.e., psychological, behavioral, physical). Upon review of Table 6.1, get into a small group of peers and discuss the following reflection questions.

- What burnout symptoms are you vulnerable to experiencing as a mental health counselor? Do you notice any themes (e.g., similar symptoms, one domain of symptoms more prevalent than others, level of severity)?
- What are some possible contributing factors for your vulnerability?
- Do you experience any other symptoms not noted?
- How can these symptoms potentially influence your personal and professional life?
- What can you do to notice and prevent experiencing these symptoms? (Self-care will be discussed in more detail later in this chapter.)

Your Agency and Clients

As briefly noted earlier, it is important to keep in mind that there are ethical concerns that can arise out of therapeutic impairment (ACA, 2014; AMHCA, 2020). Burnout and impairment are not synonymous terms. However, experiencing burnout is definitely a condition that can make you more vulnerable to being impaired. Keep in mind that impairment by itself does not imply unethical behavior. However, experiencing impairment as a counselor can potentially compromise client care, including harm. One can argue that, once clients are being harmed, the threshold for unethical behavior has been crossed.

Counselor burnout has been shown to have multiple negative effects on the agencies they work for: absenteeism/sick time, turnover, poor colleague morale, and reduced productivity (Green et al., 2013; Green et al., 2014; Prosser et al., 1997; Salyers et al., 2015; Schaufeli et al., 2009; Schulz et al., 1995; Toppinen-Tanner et al., 2005). This is concerning because such agency impact will naturally influence the quality of therapy received by clients. In fact, frequent absences and turnover have been associated with reduced fidelity to evidence-based practices (Mancini et al., 2009; Rollins et al., 2010). Considering the reciprocal nature of the person and situation, it is important to be cognizant of how your own mental health and disposition with others can influence your colleagues and the agency as a whole. By extension, this can also influence the well-being of your clients.

Mental health agencies and counselors have consistently expressed concern about the negative effects of burnout on clients including poor communication, reduced empathy, damaged therapeutic alliance, and poor engagement (Salyers et al., 2015). Unfortunately, such burnout-related symptoms have been associated with poor client treatment outcomes for depression and anxiety (Delgadillo et al., 2018). Clients themselves have also reported poor satisfaction with their care (Garman et al., 2002; McCarthy & Frieze, 1999; Phelps et al., 2009; White, 2006). Arguably, the key theme here is that your personal distress will worsen the therapeutic alliance (Briggs & Munley, 2008; Nissen-Lie et al., 2013; Salyers et al., 2015). Remember, providing mental health counseling is a unique craft. Who you are as a person is an important ingredient to facilitating client change. You cannot hide your "self" from your clients. If you are experiencing burnout, this will have a deleterious impact on your therapeutic alliance. This ultimately results in poor client care and change (not for the better). In extreme cases, the therapeutic alliance can be severely damaged to the point where it causes harm to clients (i.e., makes them worse). This is unethical.

Reflection Questions 6.1: Agency-Clients and Burnout

- Can you think of any other ways counselor burnout can have a negative influence on a mental health agency?
- What personal vulnerabilities do you have that become more salient when you are distressed? How could these vulnerabilities impact the therapeutic alliance?
- What could be some therapeutic alliance indicators that a counselor might be harming a client?

CONTRIBUTING FACTORS TO BURNOUT IN MENTAL HEALTH COUNSELORS

Although one's professional demands and organizational environment can be contributing factors to developing burnout, there are also personal traits and lifestyle habits that can act either as risk or protective factors for developing burnout. In other words, like most mental health states, there is an interaction between the individual and the environment/agency. Maslach and Goldberg (1998) in their review and reconceptualization of burnout emphasized the importance of integrating the person and situation. In many ways, the relationship is reciprocal in nature. Situational factors can influence individuals, while individuals (through their thoughts and behaviors) can influence the situation. Within the context of the mental health field, there are things that counselors can do to themselves (counselor-induced) and things that mental health agencies can do to counselors (agency-induced) that can make the job more challenging than it already is. Of course, these contributing factors do not occur in silos. Many of these factors can occur simultaneously and collectively influence each other in a reciprocal manner. This concept is important to keep in mind for the rest of this chapter.

Stuff Mental Health Counselors Do to Themselves (Counselor-Induced)

Being a mental health counselor is challenging enough. Unfortunately, there are things that counselors do to themselves that can further enhance the challenging nature of being a mental health professional. To be fair, counselors are very much human, flaws and all, just like any other group of professionals. The unique aspect of being a counselor compared to many other professions is that you have a responsibility to care for not only yourself but also those receiving your services. Furthermore, your psychological-behavioral-physical well-being is vital to providing effective services to a vulnerable population, a very rare profession trait.

Table 6.2 provides a list of common personal traits and lifestyle habits that make the job of mental health counseling more challenging (see Simionato & Simpson [2017] for an extensive literature review). Keep in mind that many of these risk factors should be viewed more on a continuum; we all have some of these qualities and engage in some of these behaviors. Rather, it becomes a concern when these risk factors accumulate in quantity and become qualitatively severe.

It is important to keep in mind that as much as external forces can contribute to the experience of burnout, a good portion of the "responsibility pie" falls on you. Consider: why is it two counselors can work for the same organization and have the same clients (relatively speaking), yet one is thriving while the other is nearly fully burned out? Of course, there could be other

Table 6.2   Counselor-Induced Contributing Factors to Burnout

Personal Traits	Lifestyle Habits
• Perfectionistic tendencies • Need to be in control • Pessimistic view of self and/or world • High-achieving • Low tolerance for frustration and ambiguity • High need for approval • Rigid thinking (black/white)/low flexibility • High internalization (success and failures) • Self-judgment • Over-identification/over-involvement (of clients) • Poor personal boundaries • Minimal humor • Mental health distress • Low self-efficacy	• Work too much • Not much relaxation • Little to no (outside) activities • Minimal exercise • Minimal socializing • Lack of close, supportive relationships • Minimal interests beyond counseling • Not getting enough sleep • Take on too many responsibilities • Stressful life events • Poor diet (inconsistent meals) • Minimal use of vacation time • Partner/family discord • Financial concerns

contributing factors, but the point is who you are as a person and how you live your life can be either a protective or a risk factor for developing burnout.

Activity 6.2: Counselor-Induced Burnout

Table 6.2 provides a list of the possible contributing factors to developing burnout. Identify at least three personal traits and three lifestyle habits that you experience, or may be vulnerable to experience, as a mental health counselor. Also rate on a scale (0–10; 0—very difficult, 10—very easily) how much you believe each personal trait or lifestyle habit can be changed. Upon review of Table 6.2, get into a small group of peers and discuss the following reflection questions.

- Are there any personal traits or lifestyle habits that you can personally identify with? How could these personal traits and/or lifestyle habits influence your personal or professional life?
- What personal traits or lifestyle habits are changeable for you? How?
- Are there any personal traits or lifestyle habits that would be challenging for you to change? What can be done?
- Can you think of any other personal traits or lifestyle habits that could potentially contribute to burnout?

Stuff Agencies Do to Counselors (Agency-Induced)

As many professionals state about their profession, it is not those that are served (e.g., students, patients, clients) that cause the most stress, it is the agency and surrounding bureaucracy. This also seems to be true in the mental health field as well. Of course, as just discussed, there are personal traits and lifestyle habits that contribute to burnout. However, there is no denying that agency factors can certainly compound and create additional stressors.

Table 6.3 provides a list of agency factors that can make the job of a mental health counselor even more challenging (Glisson et al., 2008; Maslach et al., 2001; Maslach & Goldberg, 1998; Maslach & Leiter, 2008; Morse et al., 2012; O'Halloran & Linton, 2000; Paris & Hoge, 2010; van Dierendonck et al., 2001). The agency factors are divided into two categories: nature of the job and administration/environment. There are some agency factors that simply "come with the package" of working in the mental health field. Of course, there can be variation in frequency and severity contingent upon the agency, but that will always be present to some degree. For example, no matter where you work, you should expect to do paperwork and deal with managed care organizations. Then there are administration/environment factors that do not have to "come with the package" but sometimes can be rather prevalent in some agencies. Also, note that the

Table 6.3   Agency-Induced Contributing Factors to Burnout

Nature of the job	Administration/Environment
• Heavy/large caseload • Extensive paperwork • Working long hours • Multiple back-to-back clients • Dealing with managed care • Organizational/professional politics (e.g., counselors, nurses, psychiatrists) • Limited flexibility in work schedule • Time pressure to complete duties • Challenging clients (e.g., suicidal, aggressive, psychosis, manipulative)	• Understaffing • Lack of support from co-workers (i.e., poor staff cohesion) • Lack of support from supervisor/administrators • Minimal autonomy in decisions/practice • Minimal opportunities for growth and advancement • Minimal input in decisions • Role ambiguity • Role conflict • Lack of recognition/reward for job performance • Complicated/cumbersome procedures and policies • Unrealistic performance/productivity demands • Conflict in values ("moral stress") • Unfairness • Lack of community

administration/environment factors can occur in almost any profession. The emphasis here is that such factors appear to be the most salient in contributing to burnout in the mental health field.

It is possible that being a proactive employee, you may be able to address some of these agency factors, especially if you are in a place of leadership. However, admittedly, there may be some organizational factors that are a "normal," inevitable part of the job. There may also be other agency factors that you cannot change. In both these cases, you will have to assess if these agency factors are something you can accept with minimal distress or, if they are too severe, consider alternative options for employment. A final summarizing caveat here is that you may have noticed that many of these agency factors are related to lack of control and support. Research is robust in indicating that counselors who feel like they have little or no control over their job while receiving minimal support are at a high risk for developing burnout (Lee et al., 2011; Rupert et al., 2015). Keep this in mind in your current job and while pursuing future jobs. Some environments are simply toxic and must be avoided for your own well-being.

Reflection Questions 6.2: Agency-Induced Burnout

- Are there any nature-of-the-job factors that do not sit well with you? How do your personal traits and lifestyle habits influence your perspective?
- What administration/environment factors would be a strong indicator for you to pursue working for another agency?
- What agency factors do you think you could accept (within reason) without causing much personal distress?
- What agency factors do you think are changeable?
- Can you think of any other agency factors that could potentially contribute to burnout?

MENTAL HEALTH COUNSELOR SELF-AWARENESS AND SELF-MONITORING

Now that you have read about the presentation of burnout, the possible effects of burnout on you and your clients, and contributing factors to burnout, you may be thinking, "I don't want that to happen to me!" Well, it does not have to, especially if you are able to be self-aware of your own thoughts, feelings, behaviors, and surrounding environment. It can also help to develop your own proactive self-care plan. Norcross and Vanden-Bos (2018) argue that focusing on burnout prevention is not as effective as fostering your own self-care. This is a valid point. It is possible to be cognizant of the effects and warning signs of burnout while also having a proactive self-care plan that is naturally integrated into your own daily life. In other words, it should not be something you resort to reactively when feeling distressed. Rather, it should be something that is already in place to hopefully reduce the frequency and severity of distress, in both your personal and professional life.

Ironically, while most mental health counselors have chosen a field of practice dedicated to the well-being of others, many often do not follow through on their own self-care. Stated differently, counselors do not always necessarily practice what they preach. To be fair, just like your clients, you have your own weaknesses. You are human, after all. Sometimes so much energy is put into caring for your clients (and perhaps your own family and friends) that it is hard to recognize the lack of self-care you provide for yourself. Eventually, it becomes increasingly difficult to care for others if you are unable to adequately care for yourself. Ultimately, counselor self-care is an ethical necessity for client care.

The ACA (2014) and AMHCA (2020) codes of ethics explicitly state that counselors need to be aware of any signs of impairment including mental, emotional, or physical problems. Working with clients while impaired increases the chances of engaging in unethical practice. Therefore, high-quality self-care requires continuous self-awareness of one's thoughts, emotions, behaviors, and the surrounding environment. In general, self-awareness is continuous observation and attunement to your experiences, both what is pleasant and enhancing to your life and what is distressing and threatening to your well-being (like symptoms of burnout). Self-awareness allows for self-regulation, which is your ability to recognize and effectively respond to the daily demands and stressors of life. Such self-awareness and self-regulation allows for self-care practices that can help balance your psychological, physical, relational, and spiritual needs.

Interestingly, most people are generally aware when they are under stress; however, it can be much harder to notice when experiencing burnout. This may be because stress involves experiencing "too much" physically and psychologically, while burnout involves feeling "not enough," especially with regard to empathy and motivation. With this in mind, it is important to recognize that effective self-awareness requires self-monitoring. In other words, in order to truly be self-aware of your thoughts, emotions, behaviors, and the environment you will have to take purposeful steps to track your self-care, at least those areas that are personally of most concern and risk. A survey of 595 mental health professionals ranked maintaining "self-awareness/self-monitoring" as the second highest career-sustaining behavior (Rupert & Kent, 2007). In many ways, this is not surprising considering awareness and monitoring of clients' well-being is almost automatic for most counselors. The trick is to use those same skills on yourself. When done effectively, this can dramatically protect and enhance your well-being.

Finally, self-awareness and self-monitoring are important skills, but there is nothing wrong with receiving help. If possible, self-monitoring should be supplemented with objective and validated measures (e.g., MBI; Maslach et al., 2016). Although this may seem a bit extreme at first, there can be benefits to the occasional self-assessment of burnout (e.g., standardized tracking of scores, less prone to be defensive). Certainly, your colleagues and supervisors can provide good, honest feedback. They see you in your day-to-day work activities and know your personal baseline. If you stray from your baseline, your colleagues will be the first to notice. Naturally, there is a tendency to be defensive over our own insecurities, but over time this can fade and result in a stronger sense of self. Lastly, those that are closest to us, family and friends, can provide the best feedback. Not only do they know our baseline, they also know some of our biggest flaws and deepest insecurities. If you have the courage to receive feedback from those who know you the best, you will have greatly enhanced self-awareness and overall well-being.

Activity 6.3: Self-Awareness and Self-Monitoring

Table 6.4 is a self-awareness and self-monitoring form that can be used to identify your own counselor-induced and agency-induced risk factors. Thereafter, you can indicate any of those risk factors that are most concerning to your well-being. Next, explain how these risk factors are impacting your personal life and professional life. Finally, consider what risk factors can be changed and how this can be done. If you completed some of the earlier discussion questions, you may notice some similarities in content. This is purposeful. The goal here is to experience the process of writing down your answers to "see it and feel it." Another option is to consider asking for feedback from your colleagues, family, or friends. Be sure to process your thoughts and feelings about this activity, as this experience will be important for the next two activities, which focus on identifying self-care strategies and self-monitoring.

Table 6.4   Self-Awareness and Self-Monitoring Form

1. Identify current or possible burnout risk factors.

Counselor-Induced		Agency-Induced	
Personal Traits	Lifestyle Habits	Nature of Job	Administration/Environment

2. Put an "*" next to any risk factors that are most concerning to you.
3. How are these risk factors impacting your *personal life*?

_____

_____

_____

4. How are these risk factors impacting your *professional life*?

_____

_____

_____

5. What risk factors can be changed? How?

_____

_____

_____

6. Consider asking for feedback from your colleagues, family, or friends.

_____

_____

_____

MENTAL HEALTH COUNSELOR PROACTIVE SELF-CARE STRATEGIES

Thus far, not much has been said about specific self-care strategies. Look at self-awareness and self-monitoring as a necessary initial process to foster the effectiveness of your self-care strategies. The following highlights some of the more common effective strategies for mental health counselors. Some research has referred to these strategies as "career-sustaining behaviors" (CSBs), which have been associated with positive personal and professional quality of life factors (Lawson & Myers, 2011; Stevanovic & Rupert, 2004). With that said, please do not let this review limit your own additional ideas for self-care. You know what is best for you. Just be sure that whatever you do is made a priority, something that is naturally integrated into your day-to-day activities as a life-long commitment, not a separate adjunct that will only be temporarily used. Also, when reasonable, try to initially build off your strengths and do what makes you feel most comfortable. Thereafter, begin working toward particular self-care strategies that might be outside your realm of comfort. Be mindful to not do too many new self-care strategies at once. Your life is already busy. You do not want your self-care plan to make you more distressed! The following are eight self-care domains to help inspire your self-care strategies.

Active and Healthy Body

These self-care strategies focus on the physical needs of your body, including proper exercise, diet, and sleep. Taking care of your body is obviously important for having an active and healthy mind, including overall psychological well-being. Being physically active, eating healthy, and proper sleep hygiene all greatly contribute to high energy levels and build resilience in the face of life and job stressors.

Exercise Well

Counselors spend a good portion of their day sitting in a chair, doing either therapy or paperwork. Although the job of a counselor is highly verbal, it is largely nonphysical with minimal movement. A sedentary job and lifestyle is associated with obesity, diabetes, and cardiovascular disease, which can lead to premature mortality (Thorp et al., 2011). Thus, it is not an exaggeration to state that every counselor should put a strong effort into including exercise in their weekly schedule. Physical activity is important for the body and the mind. The type of exercise truly depends on your needs. Broad examples of exercise include any type of outdoor physical activity (e.g., walking, jogging, cycling, mountain biking, hiking), spin or yoga class, swimming, lifting weights, or recreational sports (e.g., tennis, racquetball, handball). If possible, a membership to a fitness center or joining a sports league can help with motivation. Whenever possible, try to engage in such exercises outdoors. Being out in the sun and getting fresh air can also be revitalizing after spending many consecutive hours indoors.

The benefits of physical activity are wide-ranging: increased self-esteem, reduced stress, increased self-discipline, improved memory and concentration, improved sleep (quality and quantity), decreased depression and anxiety, weight control/loss, increased endurance/stamina, improved mental stamina, and overall quality of life (Pope, 2019). Finally, such physical activities provide you an opportunity to do something nonverbal. Providing yourself some silent time allows for calming down and being meditative. Or it can be an opportunity for processing recent events at the end of the day or mentally preparing for the upcoming events of the day. The ultimate message here is to simply be physically active in a way that best suits your needs. Just remember to set realistic goals, just as you do with your clients.

Eat Well

As with many jobs, when we are busy and stressed, it is more common for many of us to have poor eating habits. This includes missing or skipping meals (breakfast truly is the most important meal of the day!), eating fast food (high in fat, carbohydrates, and processed), and too much reliance on caffeinated beverages. Sometimes prepping your meals and snacks the evening/night before results in healthier food choices and feeling less inconvenienced when hungry during a busy day. (This typically results in less ordering out, which is healthier and less expensive!) You may also need to consider formally scheduling mealtimes in your daily schedule. For example, instead of squeezing in a few bites of food between sessions or while doing paperwork, actually give yourself 30 consecutive minutes to eat and relax (i.e., a true lunch break).

Although this discussion is by no means advocating for any particular diet or way of eating, there is no denying that the average American diet, which is high in sugars, saturated fats, and sodium, while low in vegetables, fruit, dairy, and oils, is largely unhealthy (U.S. Department of Health and Human Services & U.S. Department of Agriculture, 2015). It does not help that a good portion of the American diet is also processed/refined. The foods and other substances we ingest can affect the way we feel, for better or worse. If you think that your food intake is affecting your mood, consider monitoring what you eat. Try to notice how you feel about 30–60 minutes after a meal or snack. Perhaps consider eliminating and/or adding particular types of food. Also, consider monitoring your fluid intake as well. Many of us do not drink enough water. The Institute of Medicine (2005) recommends about 15.5 cups (124 ounces) of fluids a day for men and about 11.5 cups (92 ounces) of fluids a day for women (this includes about 20% of fluid from food as well). Dehydration can make you feel tired and weak, including slowed thinking and concentration (Institute of Medicine, 2005). Also, keep in mind how much talking you do each day while providing therapy and interacting with your colleagues. It is not unreasonable to consider keeping a water bottle by your side throughout the day. (By the way, it is okay to hydrate while providing therapy!) In the end, the more you improve your eating and drinking habits, the more you will notice an improvement in your overall mood and energy.

Sleep Well

Being a busy graduate student often results in not getting enough hours of sleep. It often also means having a poorer quality of sleep due to anxiety and stress. Many graduate students believe that once they get their degree and begin working full-time, they will get better sleep. Unfortunately, many of those bad sleep habits are hard to break, and the stressors of grad school are replaced by the stressors of your job and life. The National Sleep Foundation recommends 7–9 hours for those aged between 18 and 64 (Ohayon et al., 2017). It is well documented that not enough sleep and/or poor-quality sleep results in fatigue, poor concentration, irritable mood, and overall poor daily functioning (Ohayon et al., 2017). If you think that your quantity and quality of sleep are a concern, consider developing a regular sleep routine, which may require improvements in your sleep hygiene as well. There is abundant research demonstrating the effectiveness of following a sleep routine with good sleep hygiene (Irwin et al., 2006). Table 6.5 provides some of the more common steps for developing a consistent sleep routine. It is important that you follow these steps as consistently as possible for many days (i.e., do not expect dramatic improvements in just a few days; it takes time). Although these steps work for many people, they do not work for everyone. If you have poor sleep quantity/quality and these steps do not work, consider consulting with a mental health and/or medical professional, as there can be many psychological or medical reasons for poor sleep.

In addition to routine, some people may also have poor sleep hygiene. In other words, sometimes there are things that we do (or do not do) that impede the quality of our sleep. Table 6.6 provides some of the more common examples of recommended sleep hygiene habits. Most people have more control over the quality of their sleep than they realize. Sometimes just a few modifications in food/drink consumption and bedroom environment can make a significant difference in your mood and daily productivity. Regardless of the modifications you make to your sleep routine and hygiene, be sure it is a priority. It should not be viewed as an obstacle to productivity. Your body needs time every day to rest and heal, which results in greater resilience and overall well-being.

Active and Healthy Mind

As much as it is important to maintain a healthy body, it is important to maintain a healthy mind. You might be thinking that there is not much need for concern because being a mental health counselor requires having

Table 6.5   Strategies for a Good Sleep Routine

1. Try to go to bed the same time every night.
2. Only lie down in bed when you intend to sleep and you feel sleepy.
3. Only use the bed for sleeping—no reading, no television, no smartphones, no eating.
4. If you are unable to fall asleep within 10–15 minutes, get up and go to another room.
5. Stay up as long as necessary and only return to the bed when ready to sleep.
6. Repeat steps 4 and 5 as often as necessary.
7. Try to get up at the same time every morning regardless of how much sleep you got that night (set an alarm, no snooze).
8. Avoid naps (if you do, no more than 20–30 minutes and earlier in the day).

Table 6.6   Good Sleep Hygiene Habits

- Develop a consistent sleep routine (see Table 6.5).
- Avoid caffeine, alcohol, and nicotine in the evening.
- Do not eat 3–4 hours before going to sleep.
- Eat a balanced diet, including limiting fat and anything that may cause indigestion.
- Minimize light and noise in the bedroom (the darker and quieter, the better).
- Avoid extreme temperatures in the bedroom (most prefer slightly cool).
- Bed should only be used for sleeping and sex.
- Remove electronics from the bedroom (e.g., televisions, computers, smartphones).
- Consider meditation or other relaxation techniques (e.g., deep breathing, progressive muscle relaxation, visualization, warm bath).
- Read (preferably not on a screen).
- Avoid emotionally upsetting conversations and activities.
- Establish a weekly exercise plan.
- Avoid rigorous activities/exercise soon before sleeping.
- Increase exposure to natural and bright light during the day.

an active mind. It does, but having a significant portion of that activity be listening to your clients' distress and not much else is not healthy. Just like a sick body can make the mind sick, a sick mind can make the body sick. Of course, many of the strategies discussed in "Active and Healthy Body" can apply here. The focus is alternative self-care strategies that keep you mentally active outside the office and specific to your own individual interests and lifestyle. Also, keep in mind that these active self-care strategies should not increase your distress; they should decrease it.

One helpful way to keep an active mind is to serve others in an alternative capacity from counseling. One general example is doing volunteer work within your community, serving a variety of populations (or even animals). Volunteer work could also include indirect ways of helping others (e.g., building a playground or planting trees at a local park). It can be refreshing to help others in a way that does not require listening to a client's personal distress. Another example is teaching a class at a local college or university. Teaching as an adjunct does not typically require a doctorate. You may even be able to teach other master's-level students training to be counselors. In many ways, educating others is also a way of educating yourself. It is one thing to know how to do something, it is another to teach others how to do it themselves; it can make you a better counselor. Sometimes teaching can rejuvenate your passion and give new meaning to your craft.

Perhaps consider trying a new hobby or activity or returning to a favorite hobby that has been abandoned (not related to work!). Maybe you have been thinking about trying something new for a while (years!) but have not yet found the "time" or motivation. Perhaps there used to be a pastime that was an integral and enjoyable part of your life that later became just a memory over the years. It could be something as simple as reading, playing video games, or adult puzzles. Or, it could be something a little more challenging like learning a foreign language or playing an instrument. The "what" is not as important as long it is something that keeps your mind active and provides you personal pleasure.

Take a vacation. This topic could also be in the forthcoming discussion about relaxation (i.e., a mental health week, or two?). However, the suggestion here is to not just take an extended three-to-four-day weekend. When possible, it is helpful to take at least one week, maybe two weeks off. North Americans are well known for not using all their personal/vacation time. And, when they do, it is often not a full week. Of course, vacation can include rest, but it can also include adventure where you go somewhere new and different and do activities you would not normally partake in. It is good for your mind and body to get away from your office, clients, and colleagues for more than just a few days. Sometimes separating ourselves from our normal routine and environment with family and/or close friends can help us regain perspective on what is important in life.

Active and Healthy Social Life

Utilize and value your social relationships. All of us have an innate desire to be loved and cared for by others. It is well known that having at least a few quality interpersonal relationships can result in both mental health and physical health benefits. Note the emphasis here is on quality (meaningful and reciprocal active engagement), not quantity! Spending time with one's partner and family is the highest-rated career-sustaining behavior among mental health professionals (Stevanovic & Rupert, 2004). As noted earlier, counseling provides a one-way relationship. With family and friends, you are not just known as a mental health counselor (you are a parent, spouse, uncle/aunt, best friend). We tend to be most genuine and honest (the good, bad, and ugly) with our closest interpersonal relationships. Likewise, they tend to be the most honest with us in providing feedback about ourselves. Those closest to us provide companionship, security, and stability. Such relationships show us that we are valued and provide alternative perspectives outside of psychology and counseling. It meets our emotional needs and makes us better human beings and counselors. Indeed, good-quality family relationships have been shown to enhance professional functioning (Stevanovic & Rupert, 2009). As for friends, it may be prudent to not oversaturate with friends who are also mental health counselors. This provides the risk of job stressors carrying over into your personal life.

As a related interpersonal factor, humor has been found to be ranked as a top three career-sustaining behavior among mental health professionals in two separate studies (Rupert & Kent, 2007; Stevanovic & Rupert, 2004). Although it is possible to be humorous by yourself, in most cases humor is best enjoyed with others. Thus, simply spending time with friends and family with a little humor can meet two of the top three career-sustaining behaviors!

You might be thinking that currently it is not possible to spend more time with family and friends, but things will change later. ("I'll have more time once I graduate." "I'll have more time once I get my first job." "I'll have more time once I get licensed.") Or, you may think it is up to your family/friends to initiate contact. ("If he wanted to spend more time with me he would ask." "I sent her the last text. It's up to her to text me back.") Rather than giving yourself excuses or externalizing responsibility for establishing or maintaining your interpersonal relationships, take initiative. Pick up the phone and call (or text, or email) your friend. Talk to your partner that you see (we hope!) each day. There is no shame in scheduling "date nights" (or "game nights") with family or friends. Consider proactively planning breaks from work to spend time with family and friends (e.g., every Thursday afternoon, block out one hour). Try to create daily or weekly rituals to socialize. For example, make a couple days a week sacred time to have dinner with the family followed by a family activity, or schedule a weekly "game night" with friends. The primary message here is to be active in establishing and maintaining your interpersonal relationships. Do not wait for others and blame them. It is easy to take this approach when busy with work and stressed. You do not want to place the responsibility on others. It is not fair to them or you. Be the most proactive for your most important relationships. Those who are truly closest to you will reciprocate your actions. To say you do not have time or are too stressed is ironic because these are the very individuals that can stabilize and improve your well-being.

A common treatment goal for many of our clients is to be more socially engaging because we know it has vast benefits for their mental health. Does it not make sense to have this goal for ourselves as well? Our interpersonal relationships outside of work keep us grounded, humble, and appreciative of what is most important in life.

Rested and Relaxed Body and Mind

Therapy is a physically and mentally exhausting practice. Not only are you listening to your clients' life distress, you are constantly sitting in a chair for a good portion of your day. The stress of counseling and posture from sitting is often expressed through muscle tension, especially the back, shoulders, neck, and jaw. Try to be cognizant of your body posture; try to sit erect with your body straight, especially when at a desk in front of a computer screen. It is not unreasonable to consider stretching your body and taking short walks between sessions. These relaxation techniques can help increase energy and circulation. Also, there is nothing wrong with using the same deep breathing and muscle relaxation techniques you teach your clients. Relatedly, consider doing meditation and/or mindfulness techniques. Learning how to relax your mind while being nonjudgmentally aware of your surroundings and accepting present emotions has been shown to have many mental and physical health benefits for counselors (Richards et al., 2010; Thompson et al., 2014). Meditation and mindfulness techniques appear to help reduce the distress associated with all three components of burnout: depersonalization, reduced personal accomplishment, and emotional exhaustion. There is something to be said for truly having some downtime to relax and engage in personal reflection.

Consider pampering yourself a little for at least a few hours a week. For example, take a hot bath, drink your favorite tea while sitting on the couch (perhaps while reading a book next to a scented candle), watch your favorite movie/television shows, or any other activity that relaxes you. If you have some money to spend, get a haircut, pedicure/manicure, facial, or a massage. Massages are a great way to help relax muscles. Research has shown that massages can improve muscle tone, stimulate blood flow, enhance immune functioning, and reduce anxiety and depression (Field, 1998; Moyer et al., 2004). Relatedly, do not be afraid to take an occasional mental health day (some agencies provide this extra time off). Take advantage of this opportunity to get away from work to clear your mind and simply relax.

Spirituality

This can be a potentially sensitive or offensive topic to some, but it really should not be. The forthcoming discussion is by no means advocating for any religious devotion or an insistence on being spiritual. Rather, it is something for contemplation. If anything, it is worth considering where you find meaning and fulfillment in your life. If you already consider yourself a spiritual/religious individual, you may still find value in understanding the benefits to your personal life and your career as a mental health counselor. The word "spirituality" comes from the Latin word "spiritus," which means soul, courage, vigor, breath, or breath of life. Spirituality is a multidimensional human experience. For some people, being spiritual does not mean having to be religious. Spirituality is typically considered to be a force that is transcendent of one's self, including nature, the universe, and/or God. The contemporary use of the term spirituality often refers to the deepest personal values and meanings by which we live.

Interestingly, there is abundant research to support that a religious/spiritual approach to life is positively correlated with physical health (Matthews et al., 1998). These relationships are most likely due to the relatively healthy lifestyle associated with spirituality (which is not necessarily true for all people, but more often so than not). As much as we enjoy working with our clients, it can get physically and emotionally draining at times. Spirituality can be a source of reinvigorating ourselves and reestablishing a sense of well-being and life purpose. Spiritually oriented activities, including prayer, meditation, and/or feeling connected to nature, have been associated with lower work stress and burnout (Wallace et al., 2010). Spiritual resolve and making meaning out of life events are highly rated as effective coping strategies in response to the stressors of counseling (Harrison & Westwood, 2009; Medeiros & Prochaska, 1988). It is important that we have meaning and purpose in the work we do and in our personal lives. This includes optimism in the potential for growth and change in both our clients and ourselves. Living a spiritual life is purely your choice. The potential benefits of spirituality as a mental health counselor are abundant.

Professional Boundaries: Balancing Your Professional and Personal Life

It would be remiss to not emphasize the importance of maintaining professional boundaries. Keep in mind that the focus here is boundaries between your personal life and professional life (opposed to counselor–client boundaries). Some experienced counselors may roll their eyes when they hear "balancing professional and personal lives." Often, it is not because they do not care about this balance. Rather, it is an often overused phrase, and the suggestions for maintaining such a balance are often clichés and not practical. With that said, research does show that maintaining a balance between professional and personal lives is the second-highest-rated career-sustaining behavior (Stevanovic & Rupert, 2004). Thus, there must be some validity for this self-care strategy. What probably makes the difference is the specific self-care strategies that are used and how they are implemented.

One obvious, but admittedly challenging, approach to setting boundaries is not only being consistent with yourself but also advocating for yourself to your colleagues and supervisors. In other words, you first need to know your limits with your personal and professional lives, and within reason make them known within your organization. This is a must. Setting boundaries is one of the most effective self-care strategies to prevent distress and impairment (Sherman & Thelen, 1998). Admittedly, this can take some tact, especially if you are an early-career professional. Also, keep in mind that not everything is flexible; there are requirements and obligations that must be met for any job.

With that said, you may have more flexibility than you think. For example, having good time management provides you with more control over your work schedule, which improves efficiency, which means less time at work (at least not working more hours than required), which could mean more time with family and friends. You can also schedule breaks throughout the day. Understandably, you may not be able to give yourself multiple lengthy breaks (e.g., 20–30 minutes). However, at the very least try to give yourself at least 30 minutes for lunch (this means not doing any paperwork!). Also, short rest breaks of 3–5 minutes can be revitalizing. Even during a short period of time, you can take a few deep breaths, stretch your muscles, or meditate. You can even make a quick call/text to a loved one to stay connected.

In addition to time management, consider setting realistic work expectations for yourself. It is very easy to feel like you are on a hamster wheel as a mental health counselor. It is a job that can keep you on your toes in some ways (e.g., new clients with near-infinite variations of presenting problems) and can be very mundane in other ways (e.g., near-infinite paperwork). Do your best to avoid the "I musts" and "I shoulds" (make Albert Ellis proud!). In other words, avoid being a perfectionist. This may be tough for many mental health counselors. However, as you may well know, perfectionism is an impossible goal to obtain. Thus, striving for perfectionism can result only in an endless chase that is emotionally exhausting. There truly is such a thing as "good enough." Look at it this way: you cannot give 100% to everything in your life (by the way, there is no such thing as 110%, or 150%, or 200%). Giving 80–90% to many of your work tasks is often more than enough, and it leaves more time and energy for family and friends. Keep in mind, this does not mean lowering your standards or doing poor work. For example, does that progress note need to be perfectly worded? If you see 30 clients a week and you could save just 1–2 minutes per progress note, that would be an extra 30–60 minutes for yourself. In general, this is a good life skill as you get older and have more responsibilities. You will have to learn what requires most of your attention and what can still be sufficiently completed with less attention. It is impossible to do everything at 100%.

As for other boundaries that require possible negotiation with supervisors and administrators, remember that there is flexibility with limits. You will eventually have to learn when and how to say "no" to both yourself and your colleagues. (Also, saying "no" to some things will allow you to say "yes" to other things—like more self-care strategies!) For example, perhaps your supervisor asks you to take on an additional trauma client when most of your clients have a trauma history and you are feeling overwhelmed. Of course, this does not mean you say "no" to your supervisor and run out of the room. Rather, you can advocate for yourself and remind your supervisor you already have a heavy caseload, including many other trauma clients, and you are feeling a little stressed. You can even offer to take on future trauma clients after a few of your current trauma clients terminate. In general, it is best to keep your supervisors informed, both in quantity and quality (i.e., composition) of your client load and related job requirements (e.g., paperwork deadlines, meetings). Do not assume your supervisors are aware of your current work stressors and overall well-being. Your self-care is up to you. Most good supervisors and administrators are willing to compromise and be flexible if you present your position with valid evidence in a respectful manner.

Maintaining boundaries between professional and personal life also includes what you do outside your office, especially considering the recent technological advances. Technology makes it too easy to be connected to work. It is hard enough to return home from a stressful day at work without occasionally thinking about our clients. Unless required by your job, do your best to not check or answer work emails/texts or voicemail outside the office. Also do your best to avoid other work-related tasks such as completing progress notes or treatment plans (this may also be unethical if not completed on a secure network). This also includes not just when you come home each day, but also while on vacation! This not only takes away more time to be with your family, but it can also result in increasing stress levels, which affects your relationships. Your body may be with your family, but your spirit is not really with your family. Certainly, it does take self-discipline to "turn off work," but think of those who are closest to you. Just as your clients deserve your full attention while in session, your family deserves your full attention when you are at home (or wherever you are).

Finally, in general, try to minimize work blurring into personal life across all facets. In other words, not just at home, but when socializing in public with friends. Remember and respect the importance of client confidentiality. In the short term, it may provide some psychological relief to complain about work to others, but in the long term it typically perpetuates your distress and puts you at risk for coming off as unprofessional at best or doing something unethical at worst. This can be especially tempting when with your colleagues (e.g., having a few drinks after a long day). Your major connection to each other is your job, so it only makes sense to discuss what you have in common. However, try to find other commonalities to talk about besides your clients and annoying administrators. Lastly, do not post anything to social media related to your frustrations at work (e.g., challenging client, annoying colleague). This can only have a bad outcome. (See Chapter 5 for additional comments about self-awareness on the Internet, including social media.)

Mentor for You

If you have the opportunity, consider getting yourself a personal mentor. This is different from a counseling supervisor (although perhaps this individual could have been your supervisor at some point). In some cases, you could end up finding a "life mentor." This individual is typically someone who is "older and wiser" with substantial life experience (at least compared to you). Although this type of mentoring may include some professional development, the focus is more on the development of you as a person. This is a person who can help you obtain a clearer meaning out of your experiences and develop a larger purpose in life. Keep in mind, a life mentor is often someone who is not even a professional in your field: spiritual advisor; well-respected teacher/professor; wise close relative; an older, more experienced friend. Your contact with this life mentor does not have to be very frequent, perhaps just a few times a year over lunch. What is important is life guidance that this person can provide you. (The importance of finding a good supervisor is discussed in Chapter 5.)

Counselor for You

When appropriate, consider being on the receiving end of the counseling relationship. It can be an enlightening experience to know what it is like to be in the other chair. Not only can you gain some perspective on your own counseling skills (e.g., learn new approaches, learn what not to do), you can also use this as an opportunity for your own personal growth. Counseling can truly be an effective self-care strategy from the perspective of both prevention and intervention for your personal and professional stressors and challenges. Of course, you may be struggling with a mental health condition, such as depression or anxiety, for example. There is no shame in experiencing mental health distress. Being distressed emotionally does not mean you cannot adequately treat your clients. However, over time your distress could lead to impairment, which can put you at risk for inadvertently contributing to client distress. In order to provide perspective, consider that one survey found approximately 70–74% of mental health graduate students had received counseling either prior to or during graduate training (Holzman et al., 1996). A counselor seeking counseling is not uncommon. There is no shame in trying to better yourself. We are all human with our share of insecurities and vulnerabilities. In fact, it takes great strength to confront our weaknesses and improve ourselves. Regardless of your own personal reasons, being on the receiving end can provide greater self-awareness and introspection, and perhaps greater insight, appreciation, and an empathy for your clients' distress.

PUTTING IT ALL TOGETHER: YOUR OWN PERSONALIZED SELF-CARE PLAN

Many counselors find it helpful to track their self-care through broad/qualitative approaches such as free writing or a narrative journal of thoughts, feelings, and life events, while others prefer specific/quantitative approaches such as logging specific thoughts and emotions (e.g., thought record) and behaviors (e.g., food diary, exercise, work hours vs. leisure hours). Relatedly, just as with a good treatment plan, it can be helpful to write out your self-care goals and keep them visually available. These goals should be more outcome-based (i.e., measurable) than process-based. For example, an exercise goal that states "mountain bike at least 5 miles three days a week" is better than "go biking each week." Note that self-monitoring can include elements that are both qualitative and quantitative in nature. Tailor your self-care strategies to your own style and needs.

Reflection Questions 6.3: Identifying Self-Care Strategies

- What self-care domains do you think you need to focus on the most? Why?
- What self-care strategies are of most interest to you? How could these self-care strategies help you?
- Identify any self-care strategies that you used to enjoy participating in that you no longer do?
- Identify any self-care strategies that you have considered participating in but never did?
- Are there any reasons/obstacles for not trying any self-care strategies? What can you do to increase the likelihood of engaging in these self-care strategies?

Activity 6.4: Self-Care Strategies Identification and Planning

Table 6.7 is a self-care strategies identification and planning form that can be used to identify and improve your current self-care strategies and consider integrating new self-care strategies. The self-care strategies are broken down into the first six domains discussed in this section. (Obtaining a mentor and seeking therapy are unique in that they are typically not daily/continuous activities, although still important.) First, identify what domains you are already doing self-care strategies in and to what extent (how often). Second, consider what areas you think you can improve on (do better) that you are already doing and what new self-care strategies you can do for each domain. Third, identify a specific plan moving forward for each self-care strategy. In other words, when reasonable, try to make each self-care strategy as measurable and concrete (and realistic) as possible, similar to a good treatment goal. Finally, there is also a section to identify any possible obstacles to implementing each self-care strategy along with considerations

Table 6.7 Self-Care Strategies Identification and Planning Form

Self-Care Domain	What Doing Now and How Often?	What Would You Like to Do Better or Is New?	Specific Plan Moving Forward (Measurable and Concrete)	Potential Obstacles and Problem-Solve
1. Active and Healthy Body (Exercise, Eat, Sleep)				
2. Active and Healthy Mind				
3. Active and Healthy Social Life				
4. Rested and Relaxed Body and Mind				
5. Spirituality				
6. Professional Boundaries				

to problem solve. Remember, you do not have to be perfect, and self-care strategies will come more easily in some domains than others. Also, your time does not have to be evenly split among all six domains. Do what is best for your needs. What domains require the most attention will fluctuate over time. Do your best to be open to changes and trying new things.

Reflection Questions 6.4: Self-Care Strategies Identification and Planning Review

- What self-care domains are contributing the most to your well-being? How?
- What self-care domains do you want to focus on to improve your overall self-care? Why?
- What self-care strategies are your highest priority? What is your plan to integrate these self-care strategies into your daily life? Can you think of any possible obstacles? What can you do to overcome these obstacles?

Activity 6.5: Self-Care Plan Weekly Monitoring

Table 6.8 is a self-care plan weekly monitoring form than can be used to track your self-care strategy plan, including those identified in **Activity 6.4**. Sometimes it is helpful to plan out particular self-care strategies to improve adherence and effectiveness, especially those that may be new and/or challenging to you personally. Each day of the week is provided, so you can select in advance what day(s) you would like to integrate your self-care strategies. You can also include other typical daily activities and include time of day if that helps you more accurately plan your self-care strategies. If you are trying to track particular self-care domains, there is a key that provides each domain lettered. This way you can include the letter next to each self-care strategy. Also, there is the option to rate your level of pleasure and accomplishment on a 0–10 scale. At the bottom there is space to state what went well and considerations to keep moving in a positive direction. You can also identify what went wrong with any self-care strategy and provide some thoughts on how to do it differently, including overcoming any obstacles. Finally, there is space at the end to share what you learned about yourself and any final thoughts or feelings about your overall response to your weekly self-care plan. For consideration, try to begin with small, more manageable steps for each self-care strategy. Additionally, keep in mind that setbacks will happen and this is okay. Just as with any change in lifestyle, there will be challenges. Some self-care strategies will take time to adapt. The whole purpose of monitoring is to be honest with yourself, recognizing what is working and what needs improvement. You can always troubleshoot to modify your approach to each self-care strategy.

Table 6.8

Time	Monday	Tuesday	Wednesday	Thursday	Friday	Saturday	Sunday

1. Identify specific self-care strategy for desired day/time of week (take into consideration other typical daily activities).
2. Identify self-care domain:
   a. Active and Healthy Body; b. Active and Healthy Mind; c. Active and Healthy Social Life; d. Rested and Relaxed Body and Mind; e. Spirituality; f. Professional Boundaries
3. Rate Pleasure (P) 0–10
4. Rate Accomplishment (A) 0–10

5. What went well? How can you continue moving in a positive direction?

_____

_____

6. Did any self-care strategy not go as planned? How can it be done differently (obstacles to problem-solve)?

_____

_____

_____

7. What did you learn about yourself?

_____

_____

_____

8. Final thoughts or feelings moving forward?

_____

_____

_____

Reflection Questions 6.5: Self-Care Plan Weekly Monitoring Review

- Describe your general experience after completing at least one week of your self-care plan weekly monitoring form (e.g., likes/dislikes, accomplishments, struggles, thoughts, feelings).
- Was any day (or time of day) of the week particularly challenging for any of your self-care strategies? What are some possible reasons?
- What was your most pleasurable and/or accomplishing self-care strategy? What can you do to continue/improve upon this experience?
- What was your least pleasurable and/or frustrating self-care strategy? What can you do differently next time?
- Do you want to do more individual or social self-care strategies?
- What did you learn about yourself?
- What can you do to motivate yourself moving forward?

BRIEF FINAL THOUGHTS

Being a mental health counselor is very rewarding and has many benefits. There is no denying that many stressors are associated with counseling. However, that does not mean experiencing extreme emotional distress, and possible burnout, is a prerequisite to being a good counselor. The hope is that having a greater understanding of burnout and its potential risk factors and developing a self-care plan can mitigate the chances of experiencing burnout and possibly enhance your passion for the field. If you are ever feeling a little distressed or burned out and are questioning why you entered this field, try to remember your reasons for becoming a mental health counselor in the first place. Reminding yourself why you wanted to be a counselor and reconnecting with your underlying sense of purpose and meaning can sometimes be rejuvenating. Our field makes it easy to overlook the rewards while focusing on the negative events, including obsessing over failures and mistakes. Being a mental health counselor provides a unique position in life to positively influence others with your words. Sometimes this influence can result in small changes that are not always discernible. Yet, such changes can have significant amplified effects in the long term that we may not be aware of. If you are able to follow your own self-care plan, the hope is that the rewards will greatly outweigh the negatives.

REFERENCES

Acker, G. (2010). The challenges in providing services to clients with mental illness: Managed care, burnout and somatic symptoms among social workers. *Community Mental Health Journal, 46,* 591–600. https://doi.org/10.1007/s10597-009-9269-5

American Counseling Association. (2014). *ACA code of ethics.* Author.

American Mental Health Counselors Association. (2020). *AMHCA code of ethics.* Author.

Awa, W. L., Plaumann, M., & Walter, U. (2010). Burnout prevention: A review of intervention programs. *Patient Education and Counseling, 78,* 184–190. https://doi.org/10.1016/j.pec.2009.04.008

Bride, B. E. (2004). The impact of providing psychosocial services to traumatized populations. *Stress, Trauma, and Crisis, 7*(1), 29–46. https://doi.org/10.1080/15434610490281101

Briggs, D. B., & Munley, P. H. (2008). Therapist stress, coping, career sustaining behavior and the working alliance. *Psychological Reports, 103,* 443–454. https://doi.org/10.1037/e541142007-001

Butler, L. D., Carello, J., & Maguin, E. (2017). Trauma, stress, and self-care in clinical training: Predictors of burnout, decline in health status, secondary trauma stress symptoms, and compassion satisfaction. *Psychological Trauma: Theory, Research, Practice, and Policy, 9*, 416–424. https://doi.org/10.1037/tra0000187

Delgadillo, J., Saxon, D., & Barkham, M. (2018). Associations between therapists' occupational burnout and their patients' depression and anxiety treatment outcomes. *Depression and Anxiety, 35*, 844–850. https://doi.org/10.1002/da.22766

Field, T. M. (1998). Massage therapy effects. *American Psychologist, 53*, 1270–1281. https://doi.org/10.1037/0003-066x.53.12.1270

Garman, A. N., Corrigan, P. W., & Morris, S. (2002). Staff burnout and patient satisfaction: Evidence of relationships at the care unit level. *Journal of Occupational Health Psychology, 7*, 235–241. https://doi.org/10.1037/1076-8998.7.3.235

Glisson, C., Landsverk, J., Schoenwald, S., Kelleher, K., Hoagwood, K., Mayberg, S., & Green, P. (2008). Assessing the Organizational Social Context (OSC) of mental health services: Implications for research and practice. *Administration and Policy in Mental Health and Mental Health Services Research, 35*, 98–113. https://doi.org/10.1007/s10488-007-0148-5

Green, A. E., Albanese, B. J., Shapiro, N. M., & Aarons, G. A. (2014). The roles of individual and organizational factors in burnout among community-based mental health service providers. *Psychological Services, 11*, 41–49. https://doi.org/10.1037/a0035299

Green, A. E., Miller, E. A., & Aarons, G. A. (2013). Transformational leadership moderates the relationship between emotional exhaustion and turnover intention among community mental health providers. *Community Mental Health Journal, 49*, 373–379. https://doi.org/10.1007/s10597-011-9463-0

Harrison, R. L., & Westwood, M. J. (2009). Preventing vicarious traumatization of mental health therapists: Identifying protective practices. *Psychotherapy, 46*, 203–219. https://doi.org/10.1037/e695402007-001

Holzman, L. A., Searight, H. R., & Hughes, H. M. (1996). Clinical psychology graduate students and personal psychotherapy: Results of an exploratory survey. *Professional Psychology: Research and Practice, 27*, 98–101. https://doi.org/10.1037/0735-7028.27.1.98

Institute of Medicine (U.S.). (2005). *Dietary reference intakes for water, potassium, sodium, chloride, and sulfate*. National Academies Press.

Irwin, M. R., Cole, J. C., & Nicassio, P. M. (2006). Comparative meta-analysis of behavioral interventions for insomnia and their efficacy in middle-aged adults and older adults 55+ years of age. *Health Psychology, 25,* 3–14. https://doi.org/10.1037/0278-6133.25.1.3

Kaeding, A., Sougleris, C., Reid, C., van Vreeswijk, M. F., Hayes, C., Dorrian, J., & Simpson, S. (2017). Professional burnout, early maladaptive schemas, and physical health in clinical and counseling psychology trainees. *Journal of Clinical Psychology, 73,* 1782–1796. https://doi.org/10.1002/jclp.22485

Lawson, G. (2007). Counselor wellness and impairment: A national survey. *The Journal of Humanistic Counseling, Education and Development, 46,* 20–34. https://doi.org/10.1002/j.2161-1939.2007.tb00023.x

Lawson, G., & Myers, J. E. (2011). Wellness, professional quality of life, and career-sustaining behaviors: What keeps us well? *Journal of Counseling and Development, 89,* 163–171. https://doi.org/10.1002/j.1556-6678.2011.tb00074.x

Lawson, G., Venart, E., Hazler, R., & Kottler, J. (2007). Toward a culture of counselor wellness. *The Journal of Humanistic Counseling, Education and Development, 46,* 5–19. https://doi.org/10.1002/j.2161-1939.2007.tb00022.x

Lee, J., Lim, N., Yang, E., & Lee, S. M. (2011). Antecedents and consequences of three dimensions of burnout in psychotherapists: A meta-analysis. *Professional Psychology: Research and Practice, 42,* 252–258. https://doi.org/10.1037/a0023319

Lim, N., Kim, E. K., Kim, H., Yang, E., & Lee, S. M. (2010). Individual and work-related factors influencing burnout of mental health professional: A meta-analysis. *Journal of Employment Counseling, 47,* 86–96. https://doi.org/10.1002/j.2161-1920.2010.tb00093.x

Mancini, A. D., Moser, L. L., Whitley, R., McHugo, G. J., Bond, G. R., Finnerty, M. T., & Burns, B. J. (2009). Assertive community treatment: Facilitators and barriers to implementation in routine mental health settings. *Psychiatric Services, 60,* 189–195. https://doi.org/10.1176/ps.2009.60.2.189

Maslach, C., & Goldberg, J. (1998). Prevention of burnout: New perspectives. *Applied and Preventive Psychology, 7,* 63–74. https://doi.org/10.1016/S0962-1849(98)80022-X

Maslach, C., Jackson, S. E., & Leiter, M. P. (2016). *Maslach Burnout Inventory manual* (4th ed.). Mind Garden.

Maslach, C., & Leiter, M. P. (2008). Early predictors of job burnout and engagement. *Journal of Applied Psychology, 93,* 498–512. http://dx.doi.org/10.1037/0021-9010.93.3.498

Maslach, C., Schaufeli, W. B., & Leiter, M. P. (2001). Job burnout. *Annual Review of Psychology*, *52*, 397–422. https://doi.org/10.1146/annurev.psych.52.1.397

Matthews, D. A., McCullough, M. E., Larson, D. B., Koenig, H. G., Swyers, J. P., & Milano, M. G. (1998). Religious commitment and health: A review of the research and implications for family medicine. *Archives of Family Medicine*, *7*, 118–124. https://doi.org/10.1001/archfami.7.2.118

McCarthy, W. C., & Frieze, I. H. (1999). Negative aspects of therapy: Client perceptions of therapists' social influence, burnout, and quality of care. *Journal of Social Issues*, *55*, 33–50. https://doi.org/10.1111/0022-4537.00103

Medeiros, M. E., & Prochaska, J. O. (1988). Coping strategies that psychotherapists use in working with stressful clients. *Professional Psychology: Research and Practice*, *19*, 112–114. https://doi.org/10.1037/0735-7028.19.1.112

Melamed, S., Shirom, A., Toker, S., Berliner, S., & Shapira, I. (2006). Burnout and risk of cardiovascular disease: Evidence, possible causal paths, and promising research directions. *Psychological Bulletin*, *132*, 327–353. https://doi.org/10.1037/0033-2909.132.3.327

Morse, G., Salyers, M. P., Rollins, A. L., Monroe-DeVita, M., & Pfahier, C. (2012). Burnout in mental health services: A review of the problem and its remediation. *Administration and Policy in Mental Health and Mental Health Services Research*, 39, 341–352. https://doi.org/10.1007/s10488-011-0352-1

Moyer, C. A., Rounds, J., & Hannum, J. W. (2004). A meta-analysis of massage therapy research. *Psychological Bulletin*, *130*, 3–18. https://doi.org/10.1037/0033-2909.130.1.3

Nissen-Lie, H. A., Havik, O. E., Hoglend, P. A., Monsen, J. T., & Ronnestad, M. H. (2013). The contribution of the quality of therapists' personal lives to the development of the working alliance. *Journal of Counseling Psychology*, *4*, 483–495. https://doi.org/10.1037/a0033643

Norcross, J. C., & Karpiak, C. P. (2012). Clinical psychologists in the 2010s: Fifty years of the APA Division of Clinical Psychology. *Clinical Psychology: Science and Practice*, *19*(1), 1–12. https://doi.org/10.1111/j.1468-2850.2012.01269.x

Norcross, J. C., & VandenBos G. R. (2018). *Leaving it at the office: A guide to psychotherapist self-care*. Guilford Press.

O'Halloran, T. M., & Linton, J. M. (2000). Stress on the job: Self-care resources for mental health professionals. *Journal of Mental Health Counseling*, *22*, 354–364.

Ohayon, M., Wickwire, E. M., Hirshkowitz, M., Albert, S. M., Avidan, A., Daly, F. J., Dauvilliers, Y., Ferri, R., Fung, C., Gozal, D., Hazen, N., Krystal, A., Lichstein, K., Mallampalli, M., Plazzi, G., Rawding R., Scheer, F. A., Somers, V., & Vitiello, M. V. (2017). National Sleep Foundation's sleep quality recommendations: First report. *Sleep Health*, *3*, 6–19. https://doi.org/10.1016/j.sleh.2016.11.006

Paris, M., & Hoge, M. A. (2010). Burnout in the mental health workforce: A review. *Journal of Behavioral Health Services and Research*, *37*, 519–528. https://doi.org/10.1007/s11414-009-9202-2

Peterson, U., Demerouti, E., Bergström, G., Samuelsson, M., Åsberg, M., & Nygren, A. (2008). Burnout and physical and mental health among Swedish healthcare workers. *Journal of Advanced Nursing*, *62*, 84–95. https://doi.org/10.1111/j.1365-2648.2007.04580.x

Phelps, A., Lloyd, D., Creamer, M., & Forbes, D. (2009). Caring for carers in the aftermath of trauma. *Journal of Aggression, Maltreatment & Trauma*, *18*, 313–330. https://doi.org/10.1080/10926770902835899

Pope, K. S. (2019). Forty-five recent meta-analyses on the effects of exercise. Retrieved January 20, 2021 from https://kspope.com/ethics/exercise-meta-analyses.php

Prosser, D., Johnson, S., Kuipers, E., Szmukler, G., Bebbington, P., & Thornicroft, G. (1997). Perceived sources of work stress and satisfaction among hospital and community mental health staff, and their relation to mental health, burnout and job satisfaction. *Journal of Psychosomatic Research*, *43*, 51–59. https://doi.org/10.1016/s0022-3999(97)00086-x

Richards, K. C., Campenni, C. E., & Muse-Burke, J. L. (2010). Self-care and well-being of mental health professionals: The mediating role of self-awareness and mindfulness. *Journal of Mental Health Counseling*, *32*, 247–264. https://doi.org/10.17744/mehc.32.3.0n31v88304423806

Rollins, A., Salyers, M., Tsai, J., & Lydick, J. (2010). Staff turnover in statewide implementation of ACT: Relationship with ACT fidelity and other team characteristics. *Administration and Policy in Mental Health and Mental Health Services Research*, *37*, 417–426. https://doi.org/10.1007/s10488-009-0257-4

Rupert, P. A., & Kent, J. S. (2007). Gender and work setting differences in career-sustaining behaviors and burnout among professional psychologists. *Professional Psychology: Research and Practice*, *38*, 88–96. https://doi.org/10.1037/0735-7028.38.1.88

Rupert, P. A., Miller, A. O., & Dorociak, K. E. (2015). Preventing burnout: What does the research tell us? *Professional Psychology: Research and Practice*, *46*, 168–174. https://doi.org/10.1037/a0039297

Salyers, M. P., Fukui, S., Rollins, A. L., Firmin, R., Gearhart, T., Noll, J. P., Williams, S., & Davis, C. J. (2015). Burnout and self-reported quality of care in community mental health. *Administration and Policy in Mental Health and Mental Health Services Research, 42*, 61–69. https://doi.org/10.1007/s10488-014-0544-6

Schaufeli, W. B., Bakker, A. B., & van Rhenen, W. (2009). How changes in job demands and resources predict burnout, work engagement, and sickness absenteeism. *Journal of Organizational Behavior, 30*, 893–917. https://doi.org/10.1002/job.595

Schulz, R., Greenley, J. R., & Brown, R. (1995). Organization, management, and client effects on staff burnout. *Journal of Health & Social Behavior, 36*, 333–345. https://doi.org/10.2307/2137323

Sherman, M. D., & Thelen, M. H. (1998). Distress and professional impairment among psychologists in clinical practice. *Professional Psychology: Research and Practice, 29*, 79–85. https://doi.org/10.1037/0735-7028.29.1.79

Simionato, G. K., & Simpson, S. (2018). Personal risk factors associated with burnout among psychotherapists: A systematic review of the literature. *Journal of Clinical Psychology, 74*, 1431–1456. https://doi.org/10.1002/jclp.22615

Sjølie, H., Binder, P. E., & Dundas, I. (2015). Emotion work in a mental health service setting. *Qualitative Social Work: Research and Practice, 16*, 317–332. https://doi.org/10.1177/1473325015610181

Stevanovic, P., & Rupert, P. A. (2004). Career-sustaining behaviors, satisfactions, and stresses of professional psychologists. *Psychotherapy: Theory, Research, Practice, Training, 41*, 301–309. https://doi.org/10.1037/0033-3204.41.3.301

Stevanovic, P., & Rupert, P. A. (2009). Work-family spillover and life satisfaction among professional psychologists. *Professional Psychology: Research and Practice, 40*, 62–68. https://doi.org/10.1037/a0012527

Thompson, I. A., Amatea, E. S., & Thompson, E. S. (2014). Personal and contextual predictors of mental health counselors' compassion fatigue and burnout. *Journal of Mental Health Counseling, 46*, 58–77. https://doi.org/10.17744/mehc.36.1.p61m73373m4617r3

Thorp, A. A., Owen, N., Neuhaus, M., & Dunstan, D. W. (2011). Sedentary behaviors and subsequent health outcomes in adults: A systematic review of longitudinal studies, 1996–2011. *American Journal of Preventive Medicine, 41*, 207–215. https://doi.org/10.1016/j.amepre.2011.05.004

Toppinen-Tanner, S., Ojajarvi, A., Vaananen, A., Kalimo, R., & Jappinen, P. (2005). Burnout as a predictor of medically certified sick-leave absences and their diagnosed causes. *Behavioral Medicine, 31*(1), 18–27. https://doi.org/10.3200/bmed.31.1.18-32

U.S. Department of Health and Human Services, & U.S. Department of Agriculture. (2015). *2015–2020 Dietary guidelines for Americans* (8th ed.). Retrieved January 20, 2021, from http://health.gov/dietaryguidelines/2015/guidelines/

van Dierendonck, D., Schaufeli, W. B., & Buunk B. P. (2001). Burnout and inequity among human service professionals: A longitudinal study. *Journal of Occupational Health Psychology, 6*, 43–52. https://doi.org/10.1037/1076-8998.6.1.43

Walfish, S., Moritz, J. L., & Stenmark, D. E. (1991). A longitudinal study of the career satisfaction of clinical psychologists. *Professional Psychology: Research and Practice, 22*, 253–255. https://doi.org/10.1037/0735-7028.22.3.253

Wallace, S., Lee, J., & Lee, S. M. (2010). Job stress, coping strategies, and burnout among abuse-specific counselors. *Journal of Employment Counseling, 47*, 111–122. https://doi.org/10.1002/j.2161-1920.2010.tb00096.x

White, D. (2006). The hidden costs of caring: What managers need to know. *Health Care Manager, 25*, 341–347. https://doi.org/10.1097/00126450-200610000-00010

Wise, E. H., Hersh, M. A., & Gibson, C. M. (2012). Ethics, self-care, and well-being for psychologists: Reenvisioning the stress-distress continuum. *Professional Psychology: Research and Practice, 43*, 487–494. https://doi.org/10.1037/a0029446

Zapf, D., Seifer, C., Schmutte, B., Mertini, H., & Holz, M. (2001). Emotion work and job stressors and their effects on burnout. *Psychology and Health, 16*, 527–545. https://doi.org/10.1080/08870440108405525

ADDITIONAL RESOURCES

Bamonti, P. M., Keelan, C. M., Larson, N., Mentrikoski, J. M., Randall, C. L., Sly, S. K., & McNeil, D. W. (2014). Promoting ethical behavior by cultivating a culture of self-care during graduate training: A call to action. *Training and Education in Professional Psychology, 8*, 253–260. https://doi.org/10.1037/tep0000056

Baum, N. (2016). Therapist self-care to mitigate secondary traumatization. In S. Maltzman (Ed.), *The Oxford handbook of treatment processes and outcomes in psychology: A multidisciplinary, biopsychosocial approach* (pp. 136–145). Oxford University Press.

Bush, A. D. (2015). *Simple self-care for therapists: Restorative practices to weave through your workday*. W. W. Norton & Co.

Corey, G., Muratori, M., Austin, J. T., & Austin, J. A. (2018). *Counselor self-care*. American Counseling Association.

Dang, Y., & Sangganjanavanich, V. F. (2015). Promoting counselor professional and personal well-being through advocacy. *Journal of Counselor Leadership and Advocacy, 2*, 1–13. https://doi.org/10.10 80/2326716X.2015.1007179

Dorian, M., & Killebrew, J. E. (2014). A study of mindfulness and self-care: A path to self compassion for female therapists in training. *Women and Therapy, 37*(1–2), 155–163. https://doi.org/10.1080/02 703149.2014.850345

Gutierrez, D., & Mullen, P. R. (2016). Emotional intelligence and the counselor: Examining the relationship of trait emotional intelligence to counselor burnout. *Journal of Mental Health Counseling, 38*, 187–200. https://doi.org/10.17744/mehc.38.3.01

Hensel, J. M., Ruiz, C., Finney, C., & Dewa, C. S. (2015). Meta-analysis of risk factors for secondary traumatic stress in therapeutic work with trauma victims. *Journal of Traumatic Stress, 28*, 83–91. https://doi.org/10.1002/jts.21998

Hughes, G. (2014). *Competence and self-care in counselling and psychotherapy*. Routledge/Taylor & Francis Group.

Lawson, G., & Cook, J. M. (2017). Wellness, self-care, and burnout prevention. In J. S. Scott & C. S. Cashwell (eds.), *Clinical mental health counseling: Elements of effective practice* (pp. 313–335). Sage.

Malinowski, A. J. (2014). *Self-care for the mental health practitioner: The theory, research, and practice of preventing and addressing the occupational hazards of the profession*. Jessica Kingsley Publishers.

Maslach Burnout Inventory (MBI) assessment website: https://www.mindgarden.com/117-maslach-burnout-inventory-mbi

Riggar, T. F. (2016). Counselor burnout. In I. Marini & M. A. Stebnicki (eds.), *The professional counselor's desk reference* (pp. 555–558). Springer.

Shapiro, S. L., & Carlson, L. E. (2017). Mindfulness and self-care for the clinician. In S. L. Shapiro & L. E. Carlson (Eds.), *The art and science of mindfulness: Integrating mindfulness into psychology and the helping professions* (pp. 115–126). American Psychological Association.

Skovholt, Thomas M., and Trotter-Mathison, Michelle J. (2014). *The resilient practitioner: Burnout prevention and self-care strategies for counselors, therapists, teachers, and health professionals*. Routledge.

7

Developing and Expanding Your Counseling Skills

■ ■ ■

It is good to be a competent mental health counselor. It is also good to remain competent over time. Like all professions, it is vital that you continuously develop your skills and gain further insight into your practice and yourself. You do not want to become stagnant. It is considered unethical not to have a grounded theoretical orientation to govern your counseling skills (ACA, 2014; AMHCA, 2020). However, regardless of your theoretical orientation, your effectiveness is linked to your level of competence. You have an ethical responsibility to monitor your effectiveness and build upon your skills when necessary. It is impossible for you to be an expert in every area of counseling. Nevertheless, you must be competent with the presenting problems and clients that you serve. You are morally and ethically obligated to provide the best care you can for all of your clients. This will not happen if your professional development and personal growth end after you graduate. Your training has only just begun. If fact, once working full-time as a counselor is when your skills really begin to develop and evolve. However, the quality of development is determined by how much you put a conscientious effort into developing your skills. Your training and development should continue indefinitely until you are no longer in the profession. The following identifies fundamental core professional and personal areas to ensure that you are continually developing and maintaining your counseling competency.

PRACTICE WHAT YOU PREACH

It is important for counselors to practice what they preach. In other words, part of being a competent counselor goes beyond enhancing your in-session skills. It also includes practicing your counseling skills on yourself.

It may not be practical to try to utilize every technique on yourself, but there are still plenty of techniques or ways of viewing yourself/others/world that can be naturally incorporated into your lifestyle. Practicing the techniques you use with your clients on yourself can also enhance your self-awareness and insight. Not only can this foster your own skill competency, it can also enhance empathy for your clients. If it helps, consider some techniques you currently use with your clients (e.g., muscle relaxation, mindfulness, acceptance, exposure to fears, challenge negative thoughts). Is it possible that some of these techniques could enhance your own personal life? Does it not make sense to walk your talk and practice in your own life? Personal needs and ways of coping and functioning vary greatly for each individual. Perhaps you could try to integrate particular techniques into your day-to-day life (e.g., mindfulness) while other techniques may be more appropriate when you are distressed (e.g., challenge negative thoughts). Overall, practicing what you preach provides congruence and genuineness with both yourself and your clients (they do notice!). As you are hopefully aware, you cannot be your own counselor. Although it is helpful to utilize your own counseling skills for daily stressors, it is best to seek help from another mental health professional if you are experiencing significant distress.

If you have difficulty practicing the techniques you use with your clients on yourself, take some time for serious introspection. Is it because you are not sure how to apply it to yourself or because you think it is "stupid" or "won't work" on you? If it is the former, this may be a valid concern. This could be due to the pragmatics of the technique or a lack of confidence in one's skills. Either way, this could be an opportunity for personal and professional growth, ultimately benefitting your clients. If it is the latter, this could be a possible area of concern. If you struggle to see the benefits of practicing these techniques on yourself, then why use them on your clients? Furthermore, your disdain for and trepidation about the ineffectiveness of particular techniques will eventually be observed by your clients. This can come off as disingenuous and reduce therapeutic rapport and treatment effectiveness.

Reflection Questions 7.1: Practicing Client Techniques on Yourself

- What are your thoughts and feelings about using the same techniques on yourself as your clients?
- What techniques could you use on yourself? How would these techniques be helpful to you?
- What techniques would be challenging to use on yourself? Explain.

CONSIDER COUNSELING FOR YOURSELF

If reasonable, consider being on the receiving end of counseling. Do not force yourself to receive counseling if you truly do not think it is necessary. However, if you are experiencing significant distress and using some of your own counseling techniques on yourself is not working to the desired degree, then there is no shame in seeking your own mental health professional. (Counseling might be a good option if you are a graduate student!) At some point in your life it is a good idea to know what it is like to sit in the client's chair. Most mental health professionals (87%) across many disciplines (e.g., counselors, social workers, psychologists, psychiatrists) report receiving personal therapy (Orlinsky et al., 2011). In fact, the majority of mental health counselors have experienced receiving therapy with 90% reporting satisfaction and positive outcomes (Geller et al., 2005). Being a client will give you insight into what interpersonal and intervention skills you find helpful and do not find helpful, including both common factors and factors specific to particular theoretical orientations. Receiving counseling can greatly enhance your awareness of your counseling approach, resulting in modifications that improve your own interpersonal and intervention skills. You are also likely to have a sense of increased empathy, patience, and tolerance for your clients across multiple domains (Norcross, 2005), especially for disclosing personal information and modifying life habits. Personal therapy can enhance self-efficacy of your counseling skills while improving therapeutic alliance skills and agreement with clients on treatment goals and interventions (Astrand & Sandell, 2019; Gold & Hilsenroth, 2009; Probst, 2015). Overall, the more you can resolve your own personal issues and develop skills to manage your distress, the more you can help clients resolve their own personal issues and manage their distress (recall self-care discussed in Chapter 6).

If you think it is shameful or makes you less of a person to seek counseling, this also requires some introspection. Seriously consider your personal reasons for such aversion. What does this say about how you view your clients or yourself? If you have genuine disdain for those who seek counseling ("only weak people ask others for help"), your clients will definitely pick up on this as it will influence the lens of how you view others. It might be wise to consult your supervisor or a trusted colleague (or even your own counselor) to help work through these thoughts and feelings.

Reflection Questions 7.2: Sitting in the Other Chair

- What are your thoughts about considering being a client with another mental health professional? What would be most beneficial to you from this experience?

- How do you think being a client could be helpful in enhancing your empathy toward clients and use of relationship and intervention skills?
- Do you think it is shameful to be a mental health counselor and seek therapy from another mental health professional? Explain your thoughts.

PREACH WHAT YOU (CLAIM TO) PRACTICE

One obvious, but overlooked, way for counselors to develop their skills learned in graduate school is to actually apply their training with clients. Sometimes beginning counselors feel insecure about developing their skills and get so overwhelmed with their new job and its obligations that counseling ends up being "just going through the motions." Your first few years post-graduation is the most crucial time to begin applying and developing your counseling skills. You want to make sure that you secure a solid foundation in your trained theoretical orientation. Ideally, this also includes having a supervisor trained in your theoretical orientation as well (discussed in the next section). A good supervisor will help you confront your anxieties (i.e., exposure) and help you manage the other stressors that come with the job of a mental health counselor. Continuous practice and application is the most effective approach for long-term learning. The longer you go through the motions, the harder it will be to re-center yourself toward an evidence-based theoretical orientation. This is not good for your clients or the profession.

Reflection Questions 7.3: Doing What You Were Trained to Do

- What counseling techniques are you the most anxious to try with your clients? What are some reasons for your anxiety?
- What could you do to confront and overcome your anxiety to use particular counseling techniques?
- What counseling techniques do you already feel comfortable using with your clients? What makes using these techniques "easier" relative to those that you are anxious to use?

RECEIVE HIGH-QUALITY SUPERVISION

Beginning with your practicum and internship, do your best to not overlook the importance of a high-quality supervisor. Quality supervision is a key way to ensure you continue practicing the counseling skills you learned in graduate school while applying new skills as well. You want a supervisor who is nurturing and supportive while also skilled at challenging you to improve your counseling skills and personal development. A good supervisor has many of the same qualities as a good counselor and teacher: empathic, flexible, open, nonjudgmental, accepting, genuine, respectful, caring, sensitive, patient, reliable, collaborative, inquisitive, helpful, confident, supportive, and challenging (Wilson et al., 2015). They should also be comfortable with authority and evaluation and self-aware of their own strengths and limitations. As briefly noted earlier, it is also highly suggested that you obtain a supervisor who is competent in your theoretical orientation. This will not only make for a quality supervisory relationship, but also allow you to truly develop evidence-based interventions, perhaps at an expert level over time. Ideally, you want a good model for professional clinical mental health counseling.

It is easy for some beginning counselors to gravitate toward a laid-back, no-worries, "do whatever feels right from your gut" supervisor because they appear to put less pressure on you. A bad supervisor has particular qualities that can negatively affect your personal and professional development and client care: non-empathic, uncommitted, inconsistent, impatient, unproductive, preoccupied with self, and late (Wilson et al., 2015). Avoid these types of supervisors at all cost! At first, these individuals may reduce your anxiety with their laid-back approach, but in the long run you will learn very little and experience much higher anxiety. Yes, you do want a personality that is supportive. But, being supportive does not preclude being reliable and competent. It is beneficial to your professional development to be challenged. It is also beneficial to feel uncomfortable at times. It is essential to expand your independence. It is also essential to experience insightful introspection. Overall, it is vital to develop your skills. Keep in mind there is no "perfect match," but there can definitely be "horrible matches." Sometimes horrible matches can have a deleterious effect on your professional development and personal growth.

Reflection Questions 7.4: Supervisor Qualities

- What supervisor qualities are important to you for personal and professional growth?
- What supervisor qualities could hinder your personal and professional growth?
- What are your thoughts about receiving supportive challenges and constructive feedback?

OBSERVE OTHER COUNSELORS CONDUCT SESSIONS

Observing both experts and peers at a similar developmental level can also reinforce skill development and build self-efficacy. It is always great to observe experts, especially when trying to refine particular skill sets. It is good for your professional development to set a high standard to achieve. With that said, your development will benefit most from observing other counselors who are at a similar skill level as you. Primarily observing experts early in your career can be very intimidating and overwhelming. If someone is too advanced, it can be hard to pick up on the micro-skills between where you are and where the expert is (i.e., much can be lost in between). By observing counselors at a similar level you are more likely to relate to those individuals and pick up on their micro-skills while you gradually scaffold to more advanced skills.

If you are confident in the pursuit of adhering to a particular theoretical orientation, then try to observe others with similar counseling approaches. Fidelity to a theoretical orientation is important for treatment effectiveness. Also, there can still be variations in how interventions are utilized within a theoretical orientation. On the other hand, once you have obtained a secure level of developmental self-efficacy of your counseling skills, it can also be beneficial to observe those with different theoretical orientations. Even if you do not plan to take on a new theoretical orientation, there are many common factors in counseling skills that can be integrated and/or enhanced in your own practice.

Reflection Questions 7.5: Observing Others in Practice

- What could you learn the most by observing expert counselors?
- What could you learn the most by observing counselors at a similar skill level as you?
- What are your thoughts about observing counselors with a different theoretical orientation?

CONTINUE BUILDING CONCEPTUALIZATION SKILLS

While developing and enhancing your in-session counseling skills, be sure to not overlook your conceptualization skills, especially through your theoretical orientation. The effectiveness of your interventions is dependent upon the strength of your case formulation and treatment plan. Ideally, your case formulation, treatment plan, and interventions should all be consistently grounded in your theoretical orientation. Your counseling skills will have little value if your clients' presenting problems are not accurately assessed and conceptualized. Take advantage of your supervision by asking for feedback on the theoretical soundness of your case formulations. You can also ask for feedback from other colleagues familiar with your theoretical orientation. Additionally, many mental health agencies require that you revise your case formulation and treatment plan every three months. This is a great opportunity to monitor how your case conceptualization skills evolve over time.

Reflection Questions 7.6: Conceptualizing Clients' Presenting Problems

- How does conceptualizing your clients' problems help guide your treatment goals and interventions?
- What conceptualization skills are the most challenging for you?
- What could be good indicators that your conceptualization skills are improving over time?

CONTINUE FORMAL TRAINING AFTER GRADUATION

As stated earlier, your training in counseling continues well after graduation and beyond your supervision. Luckily, the counseling field provides ample opportunities to continue your professional development after attaining your degree and license. Do your best to keep up with the shifts in the field and maintain competence, including modern evidence-based practice. When reasonable, try to stay up to date with the literature by reading an occasional peer-reviewed article, edited book, or evidence-based treatment manual. Understandably, at times your motivation may be low to read extensive literature when working full-time. Do your best to remind yourself of the importance of staying up to date with effective practice. Perhaps pick just one or two journals specific to your expertise and select articles most relevant to your current practice. There are also many practice-specific books available that integrate science and practice while still being easy to read and understand. Sometimes having a reading group (e.g., one article/book a month) can increase motivation and insight. Recall the discussion in Chapter 2 about memberships in professional organizations. Many of these organizations also have their own professional conferences, which provide great opportunities to learn about some of the most modern approaches to counseling.

What will be especially important in your career development is attending conferences and participating in trainings, including continuing education units (CEUs), which are required by licensure boards to maintain an active license. The established requirements for CEUs essentially ensure that mental health counselors at the very least attend trainings on relevant topics related to practice. Of course, how CEUs are required for licensure renewal varies by state. The range (often in increments of three) for CEUs is 24–48 every two years or 12–24 annually, depending on licensure renewal schedules. Most licensure boards also have requirements for categories with stipulated content areas that must be included as part of your total of CEUs. Be sure you review your state licensing board's rules and regulations for continuing education. Some states provide a document outlining CEU requirements. For example, Massachusetts requires 30 CEUs every two years and has three categories. Category I requires a minimum of 50% (15 CEUs) including the following content areas: counseling theory; human growth and development; social and cultural foundations; the helping relationship; group dynamics, group process, and counseling; appraisal of individuals; research and evaluation; clinical services in mental health counseling; lifestyle and career development; psychopathology; legal and ethical; and spirituality. Category II requires a maximum of 50% (15 CEUs) including the content areas of professional orientation and mental health counselors and the mental health care system. Category III requires a maximum of 25% (7.5 CEUs) including the content of supervision/consultation, authored publications, and dissertations. Also, of the 30 required CEUs at least 50% (15 CEUs) have to be in-person training, which means no more than 50% (15 CEUs) can be "home study" (i.e., online). Note that the number of allowable home study CEUs (if any) varies greatly by state.

There are multiple options for obtaining CEUs. On one end of the spectrum you can take a graduate course or an institute multiday course that leads to certification in a specialized area of practice. On the other end of the spectrum you can take an online course, which typically requires reading an article and correctly answering a specified percentage of multiple-choice questions. In between, and the most common, is attending a half-day or full-day workshop or conference seminar. Workshop/seminars typically consist of listening to an expert (or group of experts) on a specific topic. This can sometimes include interaction with the audience (e.g., questions and comments) and role-playing of target skills. Overall, the cost of CEUs can be expensive, especially if attending a multiday course for specialized training/certification. On the other hand, online CEUs are relatively cheap and the least time consuming. (Recall in Chapter 5 that a provided benefit from some mental health agencies is reimbursement for CEUs. Take advantage of this, especially once licensed.)

Keep in mind that not just attending a workshop/seminar/online course will automatically provide you CEUs. Make sure that these trainings are approved by the National Board of Certified Counselors (NBCC), which is the clearinghouse for mental health counseling continuing education. Before a training is provided, individuals or organizations must submit an application and engage in a vetting process with NBCC for approval of continuing education, which includes obtaining a provider number. Upon completion of your training, you should receive a certificate that at least provides the individual's/organization's name, title of training, number of CEUs, and NBCC provider number. Be sure to hold onto these certificates because it is your responsibility to keep documentation of your CEUs. Many states do random audits during licensure renewal to ensure that you have obtained the necessary CEUs for the designated licensure period. If you cannot adequately document your CEUs, your license could be put on probation. Ultimately, if you are seeking CEUs for licensure renewal, it will be a waste of your time and money to attend a training without NBCC approval. Always look for a provider number; it should be clear. No provider number means no CEUs.

Reflection Questions 7.7: Continuous Training

- What are the most practical ways for you to stay up to date in your professional interests/areas of practice?
- What are some possible negative consequences if you do not stay up to date with your counseling knowledge and skills?
- How many CEUs are required in the state(s) you plan on getting licensed in? Do they have categories of content and allow for home study?

UNDERSTAND THE INTEGRATION OF TECHNOLOGY AND COUNSELING

There are ways to use technology (e.g., smartphone and tablet applications, virtual reality) to enhance learning and effectiveness of counseling skills for both you and your clients. Technology is readily available and part of daily life for many Americans (Pew Research Center, 2019). Research has found that clients are open and able to supplement treatment interventions with technology (e.g., smartphone apps; Aguilera & Munoz, 2011; Proudfoot et al., 2010). Furthermore, using technology to enhance counseling interventions for a variety of disorders has been shown to be effective (e.g., Anderson et al., 2013; Dettore et al., 2015). Technology can be especially helpful for engagement and motivation, psychoeducation, self-monitoring and cognitive-behavior change, and relaxation.

One growing area of technology use and counseling is teletherapy (also known as telehealth or online therapy). Through technology, counselors can provide clinical services through phone, text messaging, emailing, and teleconferencing sessions as an addition or alternative to in-person counseling. Counselors and clients are increasingly more open to using teletherapy, including clients reporting satisfaction in the therapeutic alliance (Jenkins-Guarnieri et al., 2015). In fact, research has shown that teletherapy is equally effective compared to in-person services across multiple disorders and across many populations, along with additional advantages (Hilty et al., 2013; Langarizadeh et al., 2017; Slone et al., 2012; Turgoose et al., 2018; Varker et al., 2019). The use of teletherapy has gained significant recognition since the COVID-19 pandemic. The CARES Act loosened requirements for teletherapy platforms to be HIPAA complaint. Although meant to a be temporary measure to facilitate continuity of mental health and medical care, it is not unreasonable to expect teletherapy to become a common modality for delivering counseling.

Teletherapy certainly has its advantages. A major benefit of teletherapy is that it increases access to care for clients who may not have means of transportation to and from appointments (and/or have travel cost concerns) but do have access to technology that facilitates teletherapy. Relatedly, teletherapy allows clients access to counselors with particular expertise that may not be available in their local area (e.g., counselor that knows sign language or is an expert in a neurological condition), especially those living in rural areas that may not be easily accessible. Counselors can see clients from any part of the state, providing access to a larger referral opportunity. Moreover, teletherapy facilitates continuity of care when in-person sessions are unavailable for a variety of reasons (e.g., communicable illness, physical impairment, poor weather). Teletherapy also provides an opportunity for groups of people to get together at once where it might otherwise not be an option (e.g., group or family counseling). Additionally, some clients (especially young individuals) prefer teletherapy as the primary form of counseling modality (e.g., more comfortable at home, or other location, using technology; easier to schedule/attend sessions and more efficient with time for those with busy schedules; good starting point to eventually work toward in-person counseling for those with histories of trauma or anxiety). Finally, the option of teletherapy prevents the loss of income for counselors in the event of an uncontrollable logistical barrier (e.g., pandemic, counselor illness, or disability).

Of course, there are some drawbacks to teletherapy. A major drawback of teletherapy is that it is not a viable option for clients that do not have access to technology (e.g., smartphone, tablet, computer, WiFi). Relatedly, the quality of the teletherapy connection is contingent on the technology of both parties (e.g., poor WiFi, technical difficulties). Additionally, some individuals may simply prefer in-person counseling over teletherapy, including establishing a trusting therapeutic rapport. Many important nonverbal cues and nuances may be missed by the counselor and client that might otherwise be noticed with in-person counseling. Finally, confidentiality of teletherapy is contingent upon the counselor's location (e.g., being physically located in a closed-off, confidential space) and on the client's location (e.g., living in a small apartment, some individuals may not feel comfortable being fully open, knowing that family members who are home may be able to overhear their counseling session).

Like any technology, the increasing use of teletherapy has raised some new ethical considerations. As with any form of counseling, mental health counselors have to be especially vigilant to ensure confidentially of their sessions; not just through use of HIPAA-compliant technology. In other words, counselors must make sure clients protect their own confidentiality. For example, a client in a public space with others around (e.g., coffee shop) may need a gentle reminder to find another place with more privacy, which may not always be possible. Relatedly, teletherapy counseling is considered to be taking place in both your location and the client's location. Although the ethics on the location of teletherapy counseling is still being deliberated in some states (i.e., licensure boards are looking into streamlining teletherapy across state borders), it is generally considered best practice to physically provide counseling in the state where you are licensed and to ensure that the client receiving counseling is physically in the same state as well. Counselors must also be trained to know when clients are appropriate for teletherapy, as well as when they are not (e.g., high-risk clients for safety). Additionally, if it is determined that a client is more suitable for in-person counseling, counselors are obligated to provide referrals (many states require at least three) to counselors within their local area. Clients should also not be coerced into using teletherapy or held financially responsible if the option is proposed for a unique reason (e.g., poor weather) and they refuse. For example, clients who are not willing/able to meet via teletherapy due to poor weather should be given the option to cancel or reschedule instead of treating it as a no-show and being charged. Finally, counselors will also need to make sure that they appear professional during teletherapy counseling sessions. Of course, counselors should always maintain a professional image, but it is easy to overlook certain aspects of your presentation and environment (work or home office) with teletherapy. For example, it is important to still fully dress (e.g., no nice shirt/blouse on top and pajamas on the bottom!) and groom professionally (e.g., hair not disheveled). It is also important to make sure that the background looks appropriate and there are minimal loud/distracting noises (e.g., no barking dog or children banging on the door).

Overall, although there are many benefits to using technology in counseling to enhance therapeutic outcomes, selection and application of technology should be done cautiously. First, similar to choosing an assessment, your selection process for an appropriate mode of technology should receive the same scrutiny. For example, not all smartphone applications are equal in content quality and utility. Second, do not use technology just for the sake of using technology. Your use of technology in counseling should be purposeful. If not, both you and your clients will most likely experience confusion and frustration. Third, be sure that you are familiar with any technology you use in counseling. Knowing strengths and limitations about the technology will result in a greater chance for successful implementation and relevant client feedback. Fourth, the appropriateness of technology used should be based on your clients' unique needs. What works for one client will not necessarily work for another client. If you are aware of these cautions and purposeful in your use of technology, there is great opportunity to expand and enhance the effectiveness of your interventions.

Reflection Questions 7.8: Counseling with Technology

- What ways can technology be appropriately integrated into your theoretical orientation?
- What are some problems/disorders that might "fit well" with integration of technology? What problems/disorders might not be as good a fit? Explain.
- What are some additional advantages or drawbacks to using teletherapy?

EMBRACE AND ACCEPT YOUR ANXIETIES AND INSECURITIES

You have anxieties and insecurities about yourself and as a counselor. If you are human, this is true. It is also okay. Try not to fight this or get offended. Rather, embrace and accept who you are, including your strengths and weaknesses. This is the most important step toward personal and professional growth. The thought of being a counselor in the position to influence the lives of others for better or worse can be very anxiety-provoking. "I just graduated and I have minimal experience." "What happens if I say something stupid?" "What if I can't form a therapeutic alliance?" "What if I make them worse?" "How do I respond if I'm asked a personal question?" All beginning counselors have these types of questions. It is normal.

As noted earlier, good supervision can help improve upon your weaknesses and build your confidence, competence, and versatility. With that said, you will have to also work on some of your own insecurities and anxieties on your own. What can make counseling ambiguous is that sometimes there are no clear right or wrong answers; it is much different from receiving a grade on a paper. Sometimes you do not see the benefits (or harm) clients receive from counseling until later, or never at all. Regardless of your developmental level and counseling skills, there will be days when you feel like client progress is seamless and other days you will feel client progress is near impossible. When possible, try to take some time to step back and broadly reflect upon your clients' status when they first started counseling and their present functioning. Often, you will be able to objectively note progress over time.

Being self-aware and self-reflective of your counseling skills is a must. However, be careful to not be so overfocused on the micro aspect of counseling that you miss out on the macro aspect, including your clients. The whole is truly greater than the sum of its parts. The more you are able to accept your insecurities as a counselor, the less self-conscious you will be. The less self-conscious you are, the more you will be able to be fully present and authentic with your clients. Concurrently, as you continue to develop and expand your counseling skills, be sure to gradually challenge your comfort zone. Sometimes the most influential learning experiences come from engaging in activities that make us the most uncomfortable. Anxiety is a common and expected experience when learning new skills. However, the initial distress you feel when you embrace and accept your anxiety will evolve to personal and professional growth over time.

Activity 7.1: Anxiety and Growth

First, consider the following reflection questions on your own:

- What are your anxieties and insecurities about yourself as a counselor?
- What are your thoughts about challenging your comfort zone? Is the anxiety and distress you experience for personal and professional growth "worth it"?
- What are some ways to build your self-efficacy as a counselor?

After reviewing the above questions on your own, get into a small group and process your responses. Although there will certainly be some differences, focus on the similarities. You may notice that many of your anxieties/insecurities and thoughts about challenging your comfort zone are normal for your current status of professional development. Thereafter, also discuss ways to build your self-efficacy as a counselor. In other words, what can you do to reduce some of your anxieties/insecurities while going outside your comfort zone?

REFERENCES

Aguilera, A., & Munoz, R. F. (2011). Text messaging as an adjunct to CBT in low-income populations: A usability and feasibility pilot study. *Professional Psychology: Research and Practice, 42*, 472–478. https://doi.org/10.1037/a0025499

American Counseling Association. (2014). *ACA code of ethics*. Author.

American Mental Health Counselors Association. (2020). *AMHCA code of ethics*. Author.

Anderson, P. L., Price, M., Edwards, S. M., Obasaju, M. A., Schmertz, S. K., Zimand, E., & Calamaras, M. R. (2013). Virtual reality exposure therapy for social anxiety disorder: A randomized controlled trial. *Journal of Consulting and Clinical Psychology, 81*, 751–760. https://doi.org/10.1037/a0033559

Astrand, K., & Sandell, R. (2019). Influence of personal therapy on learning and development of psychotherapeutic skills. *Psychoanalytic Psychotherapy, 33*, 34–48. https://doi.org/10.1080/02668734.2019.1570546

Dettore, D., Pozza, A., & Andersson, G. (2015). Efficacy of technology-delivered cognitive behavioural therapy for OCD versus control conditions, and in comparison with therapist-administered CBT: Meta-analysis of randomized controlled trials. *Cognitive Behaviour Therapy, 44*, 190–211. https://doi.org/10.1080/16506073.2015.1005660

Geller, J. D., Norcross, J. C., & Orlinsky, D. E. (Eds.). (2005). *The psychotherapists' own psychotherapy: Patient and clinician perspectives*. Oxford University Press.

Gold, S. H., & Hilsenroth, M. J. (2009). Effects of graduate clinician's personal therapy on therapeutic alliance. *Clinical Psychology and Psychotherapy, 16*, 159–171. https://doi.org/10.1002/cpp.1888

Hilty, D. M., Ferrer, D. C., Parish, M. B., Johnston, B., Callahan, E. J., & Yellowlees, P. M. (2013). The effectiveness of telemental health: A 2013 review. *Telemedicine and e-Health, 19*, 444–454. https://doi.org/10.1089/tmj.2013.0075

Jenkins-Guarnieri, M. A., Pruitt, L. D., Luzton, D. D., & Johnson, K. (2015). Patient perceptions of telemental health: Systematic review of direct comparisons to in-person psychotherapeutic treatments. *Telemedicine and e-Health*, *21*, 652–660. https://doi.org/10.1089/tmj.2014.0165

Langarizadeh, M., Tabatabaei, M. S., Tavakol, K., Naghipour, M., Rostami, A., & Moghbeli, F. (2017). Telemental health care, an effective alternative to conventional mental care: A systemic review. *Acta Informatica Medica*, *25*, 240–246. https://doi.org/10.5455/aim.2017.25.240-246

Norcross, J. C. (2005). The psychotherapist's own psychotherapy: Educating and developing psychologists. *American Psychologist*, *60*, 840–850. https://doi.org/10.1037/0003-066X.60.8.840

Orlinsky, D. E., Schofield, M. J., Schroder, T., & Kazantzis, N. (2011). Utilization of personal therapy by psychotherapists: A practice-friendly review and a new study. *Journal of Clinical Psychology*, *67*, 828–842. https://doi.org/10.1002/jclp.20821

Pew Research Center. (2019). *Mobile technology fact sheet*. Retrieved February 2, 2021 from: http://www.pewinternet.org/fact-sheet/mobile/

Probst, B. (2015). The other chair: Portability and translation from personal therapy to clinical practice. *Clinical Social Work Journal*, *43*, 50–61. https://doi.org/10.1007/s10615-014-0485-2

Proudfoot, J., Parker, G., Pavlovic, D. H., Manicavasagar, V., Adler, E., & Whitton, A. (2010). Community attitudes to the appropriation of mobile phones for monitoring and managing depression, anxiety, and stress. *Journal of Medical Internet Research*, *12*, 111–122. https://doi.org/10.2196/jmir.1475

Slone, N. C., Reese, R. J., & McClellan, M. J. (2012). Telepsychology outcome research with children and adolescents: A review of the literature. *Psychological Services*, *9*, 272–292. https://doi.org/10.1037/a0027607

Turgoose, D., Ashwick, R., & Murphy, D. (2018). Systematic review of lessons learned from delivering teletherapy to veterans with post-traumatic stress disorder. *Journal of Telemedicine and Telecare*, *24*, 575–585. https://doi.org/10.1177/1357633X17730443

Varker, T., Brand, R. M., Ward, J., Terhaag, S., & Phelps, A. (2019). Efficacy of synchronous telepsychology interventions for people with anxiety, depression, posttraumatic stress disorder, and adjustment disorder: A rapid evidence assessment. *Psychological Services*, *16*, 621–635. https://doi.org/10.1037/ser0000239

Wilson, H. M. N., Davies, J. S., & Weatherhead, S. (2015). Trainee therapists' experiences of supervision during training: A meta-synthesis. *Clinical Psychology and Psychotherapy, 23*, 340–351. https://doi.org/10.1002/cpp.1957

ADDITIONAL RESOURCES

American Psychological Association. (2013). Guidelines for the practice of telepsychology. Retrieved February 5, 2021, from https://www.apa.org/practice/guidelines/telepsychology

Bennett-Levy, J. Thwaites, R., Haarhoff, B., & Perry H. (2015). *Experiencing CBT from the inside out: A self-practice/self-reflection workbook for therapists.* Guilford Press.

Borders, L. D., Glosoff, H. L., Welfare, L. E., Hays, D. G., DeKruyf, L., Fernando, D. M., & Page. B. (2014). Best practices in clinical supervision: Evolution of a counseling specialty. *The Clinical Supervisor, 33*, 26–44. https://doi.org/10.1080/07325223.2014.905225

Capanna-Hodge, R. (2020). *Teletherapy toolkit: Therapist handbook for treating children and teens.* Global Institute of Children's Mental Health.

Ciclitira, K., Starr, F., Marzano, L, Brunswick, N., & Costa, A. (2012). Women counsellors' experiences of personal therapy: A thematic analysis. *Counseling and Psychotherapy Research, 12*, 136–145. https://doi.org/10.1080/14733145.2011.645050

Cooper, S. E., Campbell, L. F., & Smucker Barnwell, S. (2019). Telepsychology: A primer for counseling psychologists. *The Counseling Psychologist, 47*, 1074–1114. https://doi.org/10.1177/0011000019895276

Gilbertson, J. (2020). *Telemental health: The essential guide to providing successful online therapy.* PESI Publishing & Media.

Henry, B. W., Block, D. E., Ciesla, J. R., McGowan, B. A., & Vozenilek, J. A. (2017). Clinician behaviors in telehealth care delivery: A systematic review. *Advances in Health Sciences Education, 22*, 869–888. https://doi.org/10.1007/s10459-016-9717-2

Kolmes, K., Nagel, D. M., & Anthony, K. (2011). An ethical framework for the use of social media by mental health professionals. *Therapeutic Innovations in Light of Technology, 1*, 20–29.

National Board for Certified Counselors. (2016). Policy regarding the provision of distance professional services. Retrieved February 5, 2021, from https://www.nbcc.org/Assets/Ethics/NBCCPolicyRegardingPracticeofDistanceCounselingBoard.pdf

Luxton, D. D., Nelson, E.-L., & Maheu, M. (2016). *A practitioner's guide to telemental health: How to conduct legal, ethical, and evidence-based telepractice.* American Psychological Association.

Norcross, J. C., Bike, D. H., Evans, K. L., & Schatz, D. M. (2008). Psychologists who abstain from personal therapy: Do they practice what they preach? *Journal of Clinical Psychology, 64,* 1368–1376. https://doi.org/10.1002/jclp.20523

O'Connor, M., Munnelly, A., Whelan, R., & McHugh, L. (2018). The efficacy and acceptability of third-wave behavioral and cognitive ehealth treatments: A systematic review and meta-analysis of randomized controlled trials. *Behavior Therapy, 49,* 459–475. https://doi.org/10.1016/j.beth.2017.07.007

Pope, K. S., Sonne, J. L., & Greene, B. (2006). *What therapists don't talk about and why: Understanding taboos that hurt us and our clients* (2nd ed.). American Psychological Association.

Robertson, H. (2020). *Telemental health and distance counseling: A counselor's guide to decisions, resources, and practice.* Springer.

Waltman, S. H., Frankel, S. A., & Williston, M. A. (2016). Improving clinician self-awareness and increasing accurate representation of clinical competencies. *Practice Innovations, 1,* 178–188. https://doi.org/10.1037/pri0000026

Wang, F., & Wang, J-D.. (2017). Telehealth and sustainable improvements to quality of life. *Applied Research in Quality of Life, 12,* 173–184. https://doi.org/10.1007/S11482-016-9460-0

Whaibeh, E., Mahmoud, H., & Vogt, E. L. (2019). Reducing the treatment gap for LGBT mental health needs: The potential of telepsychiatry. *The Journal of Behavioral Health Services and Research, 47,* 424–431. https://doi.org/10.1007/s11414-019-09677-1

Wigg, R., Cushway, D., & Neal, A. (2011). Personal therapy for therapists and trainees: A theory of reflective practice from a review of the literature. *Reflective Practice, 12,* 347–359. https://doi.org/10.1080/14623943.2011.571866

Ziede, J. S., & Norcross, J. C. (2020). Personal therapy and self-care in the making of psychologists. *The Journal of Psychology, 154,* 585–618. https://doi.org/10.1080/00223980.2020.1757596

8
Private Practice

■ ■ ■

There is a good chance you have thought about starting your own private practice in counseling by the first semester of your graduate program. You may have even thought about it before applying to graduate school! In some ways, it is still too early in your professional career and development to begin private practice. In most states, you need to be licensed before you can do independent private practice, which typically takes at least two years post-graduation. With that said, it is understandable if you are already thinking about private practice, and it is never unwise to do a little reading and research about a potential future goal. The following is meant to be a primer including a general, moderately detailed outline of the major components discussed in the literature (and online) by experienced professionals in the mental health field. It is not meant as a "how to." Rather, it is best to view it as information to consider before moving forward with private practice. There are many books solely dedicated to the topic of how to start your own private practice (see Aronoff, 2017; Baumgarten, 2017; DaSilva, 2018; Grodzki, 2015).

IS PRIVATE PRACTICE RIGHT FOR YOU?

There are many factors to consider before starting a private practice. Although there are certainly many advantages, it is important to also be realistic and understand some of the potential disadvantages. There also appear to be certain personal qualities that tend to give one a greater chance at being successful in starting a private practice. Finally, it is helpful to know in advance about common mistakes others have made entering private practice. It is always best to learn from others who have traveled the same (or a similar) path ahead of us. Why make the same mistakes? This section has three detailed tables that organize this key content to help you filter all this information.

The Advantages and Disadvantages of Private Practice

There are clearly many advantages to having your own private practice. Not surprisingly, many of the advantages that come with starting a private practice are related to autonomy. For many counselors, there is nothing better than being able to do what you want on your own time (within reason, of course). You are your own boss. While there are advantages to private practice, there are also disadvantages. Ironically, many of the disadvantages are related to autonomy as well. In other words, there is much responsibility related to all the facets of counseling and business-related matters. The responsibilities can be associated with much stress, including the amount of time required for a successful practice and finances. Table 8.1 provides an extensive list of commonly reported advantages and disadvantages of having a private practice.

Table 8.1   Advantages and Disadvantages of Private Practice

Advantages	Disadvantages
• You are the boss—you decide (not someone above you) what you will do and how you will do it • You can work wherever you want (i.e., office location) • You can create an office environment that best fits your needs • You have great flexibility in when you see clients—you set your own hours and when you take time off • You can set your own fees (for out-of-pocket clients), including how much money you want to make • You can work with any type of client you want to (with limits, if taking insurance) • You can have your own approach/style to counseling (within limits—evidence-based)	• You are the boss—you are responsible for everything (e.g., counseling, scheduling, paperwork, working with managed care, record keeping, paying bills) unless others are hired • You will most likely be working much more than 40 hours a week, at least to start—may influence quality of relationships with family and friends • You can feel isolated and lonely working by yourself • If you take time off (e.g., sick or vacation), you do not make money • You do not receive a steady, predictable paycheck—income will fluctuate with client load and unpredictable factors (e.g., weather, economy) • There can be a lot of overhead expenses (e.g. leasing office space, utilities, marketing, office supplies)

• You can create jobs for others by hiring staff for assistance (e.g., scheduling, insurance claims) or additional counselors • You can pursue your own causes (e.g., what impact you have on your local community) • If your practice goes well, you have no one to credit but yourself—financial and emotional rewards	• You are responsible for your own benefits (e.g., health and dental insurance, retirement, disability) • You have to work directly with managed care organizations (not fun)—this ranges from trying to get on insurance panels to requesting additional sessions for clients to getting reimbursed for your services • You are responsible for protecting your practice (e.g., malpractice and business insurance) • You have to have good business skills (e.g., financial management, paying bills and taxes, marketing, website) • If your practice does not go well, you have no one to blame but yourself—financial and emotional losses

Do You Have the Personal Qualities to Be Successful at Private Practice?

What are the necessary qualities to possess to be successful at establishing a private practice? There is no one set of qualities. There are many different types of counselors with different trainings, skills, attitudes, and personal backgrounds who are successful at running their own private practice. However, there do seem to be some consistent themes that overlap with many of the noted qualities: persistent/motivated, organized, cope with uncertainty, work independently, make "big" decisions, look toward the future, willingness to embrace business side of practice, and skills to establish a niche. Table 8.2 provides a list of frequently reported personal qualities that are often associated with a successful private practice. Keep in mind that you do not have to have all of these qualities; albeit some are probably weighted more than others. When you review this list, be sure that you are honest with yourself. You can always take the time and effort to improve upon some of the qualities you believe to be a weakness for yourself.

What You Should Know before Starting a Private Practice

There are those who do not succeed at private practice and lament over what they should have done in hindsight. There are also those who do succeed at private practice and recognize what they could have done better or

Table 8.2   Personal Qualities for a Successful Private Practice

• Self-confident and realistically optimistic
• Self-motivated with ability to plan and follow through on goals
• Willingness to invest much time and money over a long period of time
• Effectively function independently
• Willingness to take risks and cope with uncertainty (including unsteady income)
• Basic business skills from finances to marketing (or willing to learn)
• Willingness to be okay with making money for yourself (i.e., not all self-sacrificing)
• Organized and keep accurate records, including billing
• Problem-solve
• Cope with chronic and acute stressors, including unexpected obstacles
• Financial management skills
• Time management skills
• Basic counseling skills, including your theoretical orientation (i.e., clients actually get better)
• Having a niche population and/or specialized area of practice
• Function long periods with minimal interaction/reinforcement from others
• Willingness to ask others for help
• Significant others are supportive of your goals
• Communication and interpersonal skills beyond counseling (e.g., marketing, public relations)
• Solid set of morals and ethics
• Advocate for yourself—ask for what you want or need (e.g., managed care sessions)

differently to make their journey easier. Table 8.3 provides a list of common mistakes to avoid that counselors wish they knew about before starting private practice. Some of these mistakes (or an accumulation of mistakes) have resulted in failed private practice attempts. Take a look at this detailed list of potential pitfalls to avoid. This list also foreshadows some of the upcoming sections of this chapter. Take heed.

Table 8.3 Mistakes to Avoid for a Successful Private Practice

• Not treating private practice as business, including making money
• Not investing enough time and money at start-up
• Not having enough money in savings for unexpected expenses (i.e., do not rely on credit cards)
• Starting out full-time instead of slowly easing into private practice (i.e., do not leave your full-time job until established)
• Choosing the wrong counseling fee (i.e., too low or too high)
• Little to no marketing of private practice
• No website (or very poor quality)
• Poor understanding of managed care
• Not saving money for self-employment taxes
• Not planning/saving money for slow periods of the year (e.g., December)
• Not taking into account health/dental insurance and retirement
• Not getting appropriate (or enough) insurance to protect the practice (e.g., malpractice, business, disability, umbrella)
• Poor billing and record keeping skills
• Poor financial/accounting skills
• Not establishing social outlets (e.g., group supervision, local network of private practice counselors)
• Neglecting relationships with family and friends
• Poor self-care (i.e., burnout)
• Not having a niche, especially in a competitive market
• Not connecting to the community through alternative, face-to-face means

Activity 8.1: Processing Your Thoughts about Private Practice

On your own, first review Table 8.1 and identify at least three advantages of private practice that you find most attractive. Also identify at least three disadvantages that you find the most concerning. Second, review Table 8.2 and identify at least three personal qualities for a successful private practice that you believe you currently possess. Also, identify at least three personal qualities that you believe you could improve upon. Finally, get into a small group and process your responses, including the following questions to help guide your discussion.

- Do you and your peers have similar thoughts about the advantages and disadvantages of private practice, or is there much variation? What advantages of private practice excite your group the most? What disadvantages of private practice concern your group the most?
- What are your strongest personal qualities that can potentially assist you in pursuing private practice? What qualities do you think you should improve upon?
- What common mistakes may be difficult for you to avoid (see Table 8.3)? What can you do to avoid following the same path as others who have made such mistakes?
- Considering the advantages/disadvantages, personal qualities, and common mistakes, what are your current thoughts about pursuing a private practice?

GETTING STARTED: COUNSELING PRIVATE PRACTICE IS A BUSINESS (AND THAT IS OKAY)

As already stated in the previous section's tables, one of the first things you will have to learn and accept while having a private practice is that it is a business. This may conflict with your values as being a person who serves to help others. However, helping others while enjoying it and making money are not conflicting values. There can be a balance. As the sole proprietor of your practice (i.e., business) you will be doing much more than counseling: receptionist, bookkeeper, accountant, marketing director, public relations director, and business executive (to name a few). The following are some of the most common and important steps necessary to start your counseling practice.

Financing

Ideally, you may be able to plan ahead and start putting money into a savings account solely dedicated to your private practice. You will need a considerable amount of money to start up, especially if you plan on buying or leasing office space. (There is no specific amount of money as it can vary greatly by practice.) It is not uncommon to consider obtaining a loan to cover your startup costs: bank or credit union loan, home equity loan, second mortgage, loan against a retirement plan or other investment. Of course, be careful with such loans because you will obviously have to pay them back plus interest, and if you default on your payments there could be major consequences (e.g., foreclosure of home). The more you can save in advance, the better. Your local Small Business Administration can help you develop a business plan, including developing financial statements, and appropriate steps to procure a loan.

Selecting a Business Entity

One of the most important decisions you will make is choosing the right business entity for your practice. The three most commonly associated with counseling private practice are sole proprietorship, limited liability company (LLC), and corporation. (There are also partnerships if you want to start your practice with another counselor, but this is rare.) The major differences among business entities are largely related to taxes, fees, and liability. It is best to consult with an accountant to help decide what business entity is best for you.

Sole Proprietorship

This is the most basic of the options. You are solely responsible for the assets and liabilities. There is no cost to establishing a sole proprietorship and it is a relatively simple process. You can report your net income or loss on your personal income tax (i.e., easier to file tax returns). The major drawback to a sole proprietorship is that you can be personally liable for the debts incurred by your practice and for any injuries/harm caused by negligence. This means that creditors can go after your assets such as your home, personal property, or car.

Limited Liability Company (LLC)

An LLC is the most common type of business entity used for counseling private practice (not all states allow for an LLC—check state law). It combines the characteristics of both a corporation and a partnership. An LLC is more formal and has more fees than a sole proprietorship. However, an LLC provides some tax advantages and significantly more liability protection (i.e., your personal assets are protected). You can also report your income and expenses on your personal income tax, as long as you are the only "member" of your LLC (i.e., "flow-through entity").

Corporations

In general, corporations (S-Corp or C-Corp) are usually an option if you earn significant income and/or a large company. S-Corps are the second most common choice for a counseling private practice. S-Corps can be a good option to evolve into from an LLC if you notice that you are making significant income, because there may be more tax benefits. In this case, you would have to file a separate business tax return along with other tax documents throughout the fiscal year. A C-Corp is much more complex and reserved for larger companies with multiple employees. This will most likely not be a desirable option for you unless you establish a highly thriving and growing practice!

Business Name and License

Although at first seemingly trivial, you will have to consider the formal name of your business along with your business license and employer identification number (EIN). You will most likely want to choose what is called a fictitious business name ("doing business as" [DBA]; i.e., not using your own first and/or last name). This is where you can consider the brand image you want your practice to have. Some states also require that you have specific word(s) in your business name (e.g., "counseling"). Also consider a name that you can buy a website domain for and will include key terms that will get ample "hits" on Google (e.g., counseling, therapy, mental health). Soon afterward you will need to file for a business license (or Declaration of Business Tax) in the town/city where the business is located, prior to the start of business. Finally, you will need to obtain an EIN through the Internal Revenue Service (IRS) for tax purposes. This number is also required to get paid by insurance companies or employee assistance programs. There is no application fee to apply for an EIN.

Malpractice and Business Insurance

Before seeing any clients, you will need to obtain malpractice insurance (sometimes referred to as professional liability insurance), which is a must for private practice. This protects you from any potential harm (or accusations of harm) that may come to clients from your counseling. (Malpractice insurance often also includes premises liability coverage [e.g., client slips on ice on your doorstep].) It generally takes approximately 30 days for your malpractice policy to be approved. You can obtain malpractice insurance as a member of ACA or AMHCA, or use another outside insurance agency. If you intend to own your office you will also need business insurance. There are several different types of business insurance. Your goal here is to protect yourself from damage to your property (e.g., fire, theft).

Reflection Questions 8.1: Your Private Practice Is a Business

- What are your thoughts about running your private practice as a business? Will this be easy or difficult for you?
- Is it possible to make a profit off your clients and still provide high-quality care? Explain.
- How is running your counseling private practice different from other helping professions (e.g., physician, dentist, physical therapist), if at all?

YOUR OFFICE

Unless you plan on doing only in-home therapy, you will need to acquire an office. This is typically done by leasing office space. (If you plan on solely doing teletherapy, you will probably still need an office space, as most states require the availability for in-person counseling, if necessary.) Another viable option to reduce costs when starting out is subletting from another counselor. Subletting entails renting office space from someone else who does have office space (e.g., one full day a week) at a cost (e.g., hourly rate for each client seen or monthly rate). If you have the financial resources, you can purchase your office space. You will not only need to consider cost for leasing (or purchasing), but also location, available populations to serve, and saturation and expertise of practicing counselors in the area (to name a few).

Once you have obtained your office space, you can begin furnishing it, including equipment and supplies. There is more flexibility to do this if you have purchased or leased your office space. If it is subleased, you might have limited options. The physical layout of your office is important, including aesthetics, organization, and privacy (confidentiality). You want to create a welcoming and therapeutically comfortable environment. Also, it is best to keep your client population in mind (e.g., children and families; adults) while remaining gender-neutral. Table 8.4 provides a list of the most common office furniture, equipment, and supplies for counselors.

PAPERWORK AND FORMS

As you probably already know, there is a lot of paperwork associated with counseling. The only difference is that you are now responsible for not only having all of the right forms, but also completing all of the necessary paperwork. Table 8.5 provides a list of the most commonly used forms for counseling. Of course, the types of forms used (and its contents) can vary by personal approach, state requirements, and managed care organizations, expectations. Although the word "paperwork" is used here, it is recognized that most of these forms can be completed electronically ("electricwork"?). In fact, online practice management programs (or electronic health record systems) are becoming increasingly popular with counselors in private practice. Not only can they keep client records and track billing (including insurance claims), they can also be used to schedule appointments and send automatic reminders. You can also save room with storage by scanning paper documents, which can then be shredded. These systems can save you a lot of time and money!

Table 8.4   Office Necessities

Furniture	Equipment	Supplies
• Desk • Desk Chair • Client Chairs (comfortable) • Sofa (leather is easier to clean) • Bookshelf • Clocks • Coffee Table • Side Tables • Lamps (with soft light bulbs) • Curtains • Rug • Pictures • Wall Art • Accent Decorations • Coffee Maker • Refrigerator	• Computer (and/or laptop) • Internet WiFi Modem • Printer (with scanning, copying, and faxing capabilities) • Credit Card Machine • Landline Phone (HIPAA compliant) • Smartphone • Paper Shredder (HIPAA compliant) • Locking File Cabinet • White Noise Machine • Music System with Speakers • Your Practice Sign (for outside your office)	• Pens (good quality; black and/or blue) • Ink Cartridge/Toner • Printer Paper • Lined Paper • Notepads • Sticky Notes • Stapler/Staples • Paper Clips • Medical File Folders • Clipboards • Business Cards (and holder) • Address Labels • Envelopes • Postage Stamps • Tissues (some clients cry) • Air Freshener (some clients are stinky) • Toys/Games/Arts and Crafts (for the young ones)

Table 8.5   Common Counseling Forms

Form Name	Brief Description
Disclosure Form (Informed Consent for Treatment)	Informed consent, client's rights and responsibilities, limits of confidentiality, professional background, theoretical orientation (may include description of counseling process), policy for responding to urgent incidents, fees and insurance policies, other related policies (e.g., missed appointment fees, availability after hours)
HIPAA Notice of Privacy Practices	Statement of how client's privacy is protected
Client Information Form	Includes basic client information such as name, date of birth, contact information, emergency contact information, and insurance information

Intake Form	Gathers extensive information from client history to current functioning: presenting problems, presenting symptoms, development history, social/work functioning, mental health (counseling) history, distressing thoughts and behaviors, drug/alcohol history, criminal involvement, current medications, client strengths, anticipated challenges
Release of Information Form	Necessary to communicate/release information to a third party, including managed care organizations
Social Media/Electronic Communication Policy	Clear explanation for not accepting friend/connection requests with clients and policy for using email (e.g., no personal/clinical information)
Consent for Treatment of Minor	Need parent/guardian consent to provide counseling to someone under 18 years old
Progress Note	Best to have a formal, systematic method to take notes while in session, including managed care requirements
Client Contact Form	Includes contact with client (or other parties on behalf of the client) other than counseling sessions (e.g., phone call, email)
Formal Assessments	Any broad-band or disorder/problem-specific assessments to help track client's current functioning and progress in counseling
Treatment Plan	Case formulation (or separate form), diagnosis, presenting problems, treatment goals, interventions (and/or objectives), client signature to indicate treatment plan reviewed
Discharge Plan and Summary	Completed when counseling is complete to indicate progress made (e.g., treatment goals completed), reason for termination, and possible referrals moving forward
Referral Form	Provide contact information of any possible referrals, client signature to indicate receipt of form

THE BUSINESS OF A PRIVATE PRACTICE

As stated earlier, something that is challenging for many counselors that begin private practice is to understand and embrace the fact that it is a business. This includes many aspects of a "typical business," including managing finances. This requires that you have a business plan, which includes knowing how to budget expenses, bookkeeping/accounting skills, setting fees, marketing/advertising (discussed later as a separate section), payroll and benefits, and working with managed care organizations. Overall, running your own business is hard enough without adding additional obstacles such as poor business skills and low motivation to accept that it is okay to make a financial profit from counseling your clients.

Learn How to Manage Finances

It is important for counselors entering private practice to begin with a money mindset. Many counselors appear to believe that private practice is not the place to make a lot of money. In fact, making a lot of money is perceived as being "selfish," "unethical," "immoral," and "in 'it' for the wrong reasons." As helpers, many counselors feel like caring for clients and making money from clients is a contradiction in values. This does not have to be the case. Providing quality care to clients while making (more than) enough money to have a comfortable lifestyle is okay.

Some people are naturally good at managing their own finances, and with some reading, consulting, and practice these skills can naturally transfer over to managing a private practice. There are others, however, who have a hard time keeping track of their finances, including paying bills on time and being able to save money (i.e., not rack up credit card debt) over time. If you are one of the latter, you will definitely want to learn how to manage finances. Obviously, if you can barely manage your own finances, you will not be able to manage your business finances. If you are one of the former, it would still be wise to learn the key components of business finances. Although there are clearly transferable skills from personal to business finances, there are many idiosyncratic aspects. Overall, developing a money mindset requires forming healthy business habits.

Develop a Business Plan

After doing some of your own research and consulting with others, it is wise to develop your own business plan. Typically, you should provide an overview of the practice first, followed by financials. Some of the most common components of a business plan include (a) introductory information (e.g., executive summary, mission statement, type of business formation, types of services provided, vision), (b) market research (e.g., number of potential clients, what is known about competition, local market trends that may affect business), (c) marketing plan (e.g., portions of the market the practice will address, advertising and promotional activities), (d) operational plan (e.g., organizational structure, how records will be kept and protected), (e) status and outlook (e.g., capabilities [strengths], challenges [weaknesses], chances [opportunities], concerns [threats], and (f) financial information and plan (e.g., initial capital and first-year estimates, estimate revenue beyond break-even point, beginning balance sheet). Unless you apply for a loan or a grant, you do not need a formal business plan. However, it is still wise to develop one before beginning a business because it gives you a foundation and organized structure moving forward. Indeed, your business is not set in stone. You can always make modifications as you learn, and your business evolves over time.

Budgeting and Financial Planning

One of the most important aspects of running a sound business is keeping good records. Be sure you understand where your money is coming and going from the very beginning. Some counselors obtain a bookkeeper or an accountant to help with financial record keeping and related financials such as taxes. With that said, this may not be an option for everyone, and it is still important to know how to maintain organized records, budget, and read financial reports on your own. You will need to consider that you have to file your business taxes with the IRS. Having an accountant will be most helpful for this. You will also have to make such decisions as whether to file your taxes on a fiscal year (July–June) or a calendar year (January–December); and you will most likely have to pay your taxes quarterly. It is also highly suggested that you follow what is called "generally accepted accounting principles," which is a double-entry system of accounting. This is a common system that allows for double-entry (i.e., debits and credits) to ensure accounts "balance." You will also have to decide if accounting is on a cash basis (i.e., income is recognized when cash is received, and expenses are recognized when cash is paid out) or an accrual basis (i.e., recognizes when income is earned [but not yet received] and when expenses are incurred [but not yet paid] regardless of when cash is actually received or disbursed).

A very important task is to establish an annual budget that details your anticipated income and expenses (often broken down monthly). This should include budgeting for a loan, purchasing or leasing office space, initial office necessities (e.g., furniture, equipment, and supplies), and common business expenses. It is important to be conservative about your projected income and realistic about your anticipated expenses. At the very least you will need to ensure that you can pay your monthly expenses—this is called your "breakeven analysis." Overall, even if you intend to use an accountant, it is advised to use at least a simple spreadsheet or consider accounting software such as QuickBooks, FreshBooks, or counseling software that may have an accounting component. At the very least you will have to be able to produce such financial reports as a "balance sheet" (i.e., statement of the financial position of the business) and an "income and expense statement" (i.e., net income or expenses at the end of each accounting period—typically every month).

Of course, like any business, you cannot forget about your taxes, benefits, and insurance coverages. You will need to make sure that you account
for all of these additional expenses in your monthly (and overall) budgeting.
For taxes, it is most commonly recommended to put away 30% of what
you pay yourself (perhaps in a separate account) so that you can pay federal and state taxes. Note that what you pay yourself comes after you pay
your monthly business expenses from your business account. Also keep in
mind that your taxes will include "self-employment tax," which consists
of social security and Medicare tax. This may sound a bit confusing when
hearing about business taxes for the first time. The IRS provides a "Business
Tax Kit," which includes Publication 583, otherwise known as "Starting a
Business and Keeping Records," along with other information and forms.
Finally, keep in mind that because you will be running a business, you will
be expected to pay taxes four times a year rather than once a year for personal taxes like most people are used to doing.

Unless you have another source of income, you will need to put away
money for retirement savings (e.g., simplified employee pension [SEP],
one-participant 401K account). You will also need to purchase your own
health and dental insurance if you cannot use your partner's/spouse's employer-
subsidized benefits. Disability insurance is also wise so you can cover income
lost for injury and physical/mental health disorders. If you have other people
you are responsible for (e.g., partner/spouse, children), you should feel morally
obligated to protect them from financial burdens in the case of death through
life insurance. Malpractice (also known as professional liability) insurance
and business insurance were discussed earlier. Finally, umbrella insurance is
wise to have for additional coverage after other polices have met their max-
imums or gone outside their limitations. Although some of these insurance
policies seem overwhelming and it is tempting to not get coverage, they are
vital to your financial solvency and protection of your assets for a relatively
inexpensive monthly cost. Table 8.6 provides a list of common monthly business expenses for counseling private practice (note: this list does not include
office necessities like furniture, equipment, and supplies—see Table 8.4).

Part of the financial process will include setting up a separate business
checking account (the IRS likes this ... so do this). Having a separate business account makes bookkeeping and filing taxes much easier and "cleaner"
for both you and your accountant. This allows you to account for your business as a financial entity separate from yourself. This means that each time
a client pays you or you get reimbursed from managed care, it should go
straight into your business checking account. Payment from clients can be
cash, check, or credit card. The most common systems for processing credit
cards include Square, Stripe, PayPal, Intuit, and EMS. With all of these systems there is a fee per transaction (i.e., swipe rate and keyed rate) and a

Table 8.6   Common Monthly Business Expenses

• Office rent/lease • Electricity/heating • Internet • Cell phone • Landline phone system • Website • Marketing/advertising • Office supplies • Office cleaning/repair • *Depreciation of furniture and equipment (items will need to be replaced over time)	• Malpractice (professional liability) insurance • Business insurance • Disability insurance • Life insurance • Umbrella insurance • Medical and dental insurance • Retirement savings • Books/articles • License renewal fees • Professional membership dues • Continuing education fees	• Bookkeeping/ accountant fees (taxes and tax preparation) • Billing/accounting software • Practice management software • Banking fees • Legal consulting • Travel • Supervision • Networking

variety of supplemental resources. Which one is "best" depends on the current rates and your desired resources. Payment from managed care can be through check, but most choose direct deposit. You will also need to pay any business-related expenses through your business account as well. You can "pay yourself" by transferring money from your business account to your personal account. Generally, money should only flow from your business account into other accounts, unless you are lending personal money to your business, which should be accounted for.

Setting and Disclosing Fees

In order to have a viable business, you need to make money. In order to make money, you need to know your "value" in dollar terms. This means being comfortable with charging a fee that accurately reflects your worth within your practicing area's market. Your fee is the primary (perhaps only) way of making money for your business. This may require comparing your fees to other counselors in your area, and even other quasi-related professions (e.g., physical therapist, massage therapist, dentist, family doctor). You will also want to review your business expenses within the context of how many billable sessions you plan on having each week. In other words, you will want to do the math based upon the context of your business expenses and external environment. On the one hand, you do not want to undersell yourself and offer an unsustainably low fee. One the other hand, you do not want to alienate prospective clients by offering an impossibly high fee. Of course, setting fees largely has to do with providing services for clients who pay out of pocket. When you get paneled with insurance providers, you will be bound to what the payer agrees to pay. Nevertheless, you will also need to learn to be comfortable asking clients for money (e.g., fee or copay before each session), including following up with clients on late payments or fees for no-shows or late cancellations. Admittedly, it is a delicate balance between collecting fees for services while maintaining a strong therapeutic rapport.

Managed Care Organizations

Unless you plan on working only with self-pay clients, you will need to work with managed care organizations (MCOs) to get reimbursed for your services. Mental health counselors have a wide range of opinions about accepting health insurance in private practice. The primary (and probably only) reason why anyone decides to work with MCOs is the steady flow of clients you can receive. In other words, although it is important to always market your private practice, clients will also come to you through their insurance provider. On the other hand, some of the more common negative aspects of working with MCOs include additional paperwork, restrictions on length and number of sessions, spending much time sorting out claims and benefits, and often lower payment fees than for self-pay clients. Depending on your location, expertise, and competition, it may be difficult to begin your practice with just self-pay clients. A common approach is to start off with accepting insurance and gradually transition to self-pay as more experience and established expertise is gained.

If you want to work with health insurance clients, you will need to get on what is called "insurance panels." Being a provider on an insurance panel (i.e., "credentialed") means you have signed a contract at a negotiated lower rate of payment to have access to their members. This means you are an "in-network" provider. ("Out-of-network" is when you see a client with insurance you are not credentialed for. This is not as common, as clients typically pay you upfront and it costs more to them than does an in-network provider.) Typically, once you are credentialed, you can only get reimbursed for the diagnosis and treatment of a mental health disorder. It can be very difficult to get on an insurance panel without being licensed, but it is possible in rare cases. Some insurance companies also require a certain number of years of counseling experience. Another obstacle is not getting paneled because the insurance company is at full capacity. Not being accepted to an insurance due to full capacity is more common in urban areas than in suburban or rural areas. You can reapply every 90 days to see if there is an opening. Sometimes you can appeal a rejection by highlighting your expertise and the necessity for more mental health counselors in your area (i.e., they will benefit from your services). The application process for insurance panels is known to be very time-consuming due to their lengthy applications and extensive supportive documents. Before you apply, you will also need to create a Council for Affordable Quality Healthcare (CAQH) profile online and apply for a National Provider Identification (NPI) number (you may already have this from your internship and other employment). Applications have also been known to get "lost" in the system, and then magically disappear. So, it is best to make copies of your application and continuously follow up on its status. There are also people you can hire to submit your application due to its cumbersome and frustrating nature. Once it is accepted, you have to review and sign a contract that includes an agreed-upon fee. Enjoy!

There are also third-party payers (i.e., not self-pay or insurance) that you can choose to get contracts with. Common third-party payers include employee assistance programs, Medicare, Medicaid, Tricare, Children's Healthcare Insurance Program, and local government programs. Obtaining contracts with such providers may result in serving clients within your expertise while also diversifying your payment options.

Reflection Questions 8.2: The Business Side of Running a Business

- What are your thoughts about developing your own business plan?
- Do you believe you have good budgeting and financial management and planning skills? What can you do to improve upon this skill set? What are your thoughts about finances with regard to running a business?
- What are your thoughts about collecting money from clients? Does it make a difference if it is a co-pay, no-show fee, or following up on a late payment?
- What are your concerns about working with MCOs? Do you think the benefits outweigh these concerns? Do you think it is possible to run a successful private practice with only self-pay clients?

MARKETING

Whether you plan on serving only clients with insurance or self-pay clients, it is vital that you market your practice. If the thought of marketing makes you cringe, remember that private practice counseling is a business, and all businesses need at least some form of marketing to survive. You do not have to like it, but you do have to do it. The days of hanging a shingle and waiting for clients to come walking through your door are long over (as in 30+ years ago). What strategies you use will vary greatly on the location of your practice, types of clients served, and your own personality/ style. One thing that has definitely changed is the ease of advertising due to the Internet. Although print advertisements still have their place, much of your advertising will be done online. It can also help to step away from your computer and go outside your door and interact directly with those in your community.

Develop a Marketing Plan

Technically, marketing is much more than advertising. How you simply present yourself on a day-to-day basis is a form of marketing for your business. This can be a good or a bad thing. Rather than fighting it, accept that how you present yourself and your business (formal or informal) will have an impact on your success. Knowing that marketing is unavoidable, it is best to at least be purposeful in your approach. Some counselors have found it helpful to develop a formal marketing plan before moving forward: (a) evaluate opportunities and threats of your external environment (e.g., competition, economics, politics), (b) evaluate opportunities and threats to your internal environment (e.g., financial standing, technology, informational), (c) analyze marketing opportunity (e.g., existing or new clients/markets you can serve, needs of the community), (d) where you see your practice in the future (e.g., could include mission statement), (e) performance objectives (e.g., benchmarks to track progress), and (f) strategic marketing plan (e.g., techniques, means of advertising, cost—time and money). Ultimately, you will need to determine your clients' needs and the best way to engage and communicate with them in order to be a viable option to provide them your services. Stated differently, you want a marketing plan that helps potential clients understand who you are and that you offer valuable services that they can benefit from. This requires an ability to articulate what you have to offer, including a possible niche for your practice.

Develop a Niche for Your Practice

Before formally advertising, you ideally want to develop a niche for your practice. Specialty niches are known to provide the best income for your time and energy. This should be a combination of your expertise and knowing the needs of your local community. Do your best to track the social, economic, and political trends of your service area. In many cases, you will be setting up a private practice where there are other practicing mental health professionals. If you can "sell yourself" as someone who has expertise in a few specific areas that can meet the needs of your community, you have a better chance of standing out from other practitioners (i.e., "competition").

This does not mean you cannot still have a generalist approach with regard to disorders treated and clients served. It simply means that you can try to sell yourself as an expert in particular areas (e.g., CBT for trauma [e.g., for veterans or sexual assault], LGBTQ+ care, anger management for teens). Some argue that having a pure niche (i.e., no generalist components) is the way to go, but this really depends on your own expertise and what is best for your practice. Overall, the safest approach is often to start off more generalist in nature (this is good for professional development as well) and specialize over time as you gain more skills, develop the identity of your practice, and understand your community more.

If you decide to develop a niche, be sure to learn as much as you can about your chosen area of expertise. This includes keeping up with the current literature, participating in trainings, attending workshops/seminars, taking classes, and consulting with other established experts. It will take time to develop your expertise. You will not be the "best" counselor for every potential client, but you can be at least one of the best for your niche. As you gain more skills and provide successful counseling for clients, your reputation will naturally catch on as being an expert. Some of your best marketing can come from clients you have successfully treated. Happy clients will talk about you and refer other potential clients. This will be especially true if you are successfully offering services that no other counselor is (or very few are) providing in your community. This will make marketing and advertising your services much easier.

"Direct Forms" of Advertising
Direct forms of advertising here simply mean a modality that identifies your practice and how to contact you for services. One of the most common approaches is to post online advertisements to various websites. Of course, online advertising is not cheap. Similarly, it is highly suggested that you develop your own website for your practice. This is where you can "advertise" your services and contact information, and provide any links related to your practice. Another highly suggested option is to get your practice info published in Psychology Today's directory (or other related online directories). You can state your area of expertise and populations served, and provide a link to your website. You can also have a Facebook, Instagram, or Twitter account solely dedicated to the advertising of your practice. Yes, you can still leave ads in newspapers and newsletters (as in actual paper). Also in paper format are business cards and brochures, which are easy to distribute and can have other advertising content (website, address, email, phone).

Activity 8.2: Reviewing Private Practice Websites

Although it is currently too soon to be developing your own private practice website, it can be fun and inspiring to look at the websites of other mental health counselors. Do an internet search of a geographical area that you think you might someday do private practice in. You can also do a geographical search on Psychology Today. There, you will find a descriptive profile, including therapeutic services provided by the counselor. Many of these counselors also have their own websites linked to their profiles. While looking at the websites, consider what you like and do not like: practice name, description of the counselor, description of the therapeutic approach and clients served, availability of counselor, ways to schedule a first session, frequently asked questions, and the overall look of the website (e.g., themes, images, colors, font type/size). It can always be fun to fantasize what your future business may look like!

"Indirect Forms" of Advertising

Indirect forms of advertising are when you post content relevant to your practice, but it is not the primary function (at least not on the surface). Ways you can do this is to write blogs, articles, or newsletters about topics on which you are knowledgeable (i.e., expert) and geared toward your desired populations. You can even write for such mental health outlets as Psychology Today or Good Therapy. Similarly, instead of writing, you can post videos (i.e., vlogs) or audio recordings (i.e., podcasts) of yourself talking about relevant topics. Although Facebook, Instagram, and Twitter were mentioned as a direct form of marketing, they can also be an indirect form by posting interesting content (either found elsewhere or written yourself) that may be relevant to your practice. Much of this content can also be posted within or linked to your website and/or YouTube. Overall, this will give you a good social media presence (i.e., good search engine optimization) as your name and practice get linked to various mental health and counseling content.

Networking

One of the best ways to get referrals is through networking. Establishing personal connections with other providers and professionals in the community can go a long way. Networking does take time and effort (and courage), but it is worth the investment. It is okay to do some explicit self-promotion with other professionals. There is nothing wrong with informing others that you are in private practice and you have some openings that you are looking to fill, especially with colleagues and other professionals you know.

Of course, there may be many other professionals you do not know (at least not personally), and you will have to use alternative means to reach out to them.

One quick way to start networking is to develop a LinkedIn account. This form of social media focuses on the professional aspects of your life. (Look at it as the Facebook of the professional world.) After developing your profile, you can try to "link" to other professionals in your community. This provides an initial opportunity to learn about potential referral sources. However, this is only a start. Be sure to use more direct means to expand your network. One effective approach to networking is simply to directly reach out to other practitioners and professionals in your community. This can include physicians, attorneys, physical therapists, accountants, ministers-clergy, educators, nurses (including school), and even other counselors. It is wise to reach out to these individuals in a personal way. Send them an email and a letter (yes, by mail) explaining who you are, what services you provide, and how you can be helpful to their clients/patients. Also, whenever possible, a face-to-face meeting (e.g., coffee or lunch) can be even more impactful. Many professionals do not feel comfortable sending their clients/patients to people they do not know. They need to see a face and get a sense of your personality. It is always important to be sure that you emphasize what they can gain by establishing a relationship with you. (It is already clear what you are looking for [i.e., more clients].) You want to take the time to learn about them and show genuine interest in them and what they do. If there is a good connection and they seem interested in what you do, then you can elaborate further on your practice and desire for client referrals. Just a few good referral sources can result in more clients than traditional advertising.

Community Work

In some ways, online advertising may not be very intimidating because you do not have to interact face-to-face with other providers and potential clients. However, marketing yourself in the community can be a very effective way to attract attention to your practice. You may not know this, but you might actually be an expert on a few topics (or at least more knowledgeable than most). This provides an opportunity to give talks to groups and associations at their meetings/conferences/events. You can even reach out to your local community and see if their needs match your expertise. You could start broad and offer a free seminar or workshop (perhaps on a topic of your choice) at a community resource center or public library. You could also contact local agencies to assess their needs: police/fire department coping with PTSD, school system trying to manage disruptive behaviors and/or depressed/suicidal students, or physicians with patients dealing with chronic pain. Not only do these talks give you the opportunity to provide a service to your local community, you can also use this approach as a subtle way to expand awareness of your practice. There is nothing wrong in telling your audience that you have a private practice while also providing "leave behinds" (e.g., business cards, brochures, flyers, or pens with contact information). As a nice bonus, if you get a positive reputation, some of these talks could result in making additional income as well. Some counselors will also sponsor local charities and participate in community volunteer work. Overall, you want to give yourself a presence in your community while being genuine in who you are as a person and a professional.

Reflection Questions 8.3: Selling Yourself (Your Business)

- What are your thoughts about having to market your private practice? Can you still be a competent and professional counselor while marketing your services?
- Although early in your career, what are some possible niches for your private practice? What are your thoughts and feelings about referring to yourself as an expert in advertising your services?
- How successful do you think you can be in networking with other providers in your community? Can you think of any potential obstacles (internal or environmental)?
- What could you do in your community as an alternative form of marketing?

CONCLUDING COMMENTS

So, do you still think private practice is right for you? As stated at the beginning of the chapter, this review of basic private practice components is by no means exhaustive. There are many more key components to private practice, and those components covered here could each be worthy of a separate chapter in a book fully dedicated to private practice. Nevertheless, this primer on private practice was provided to at least get you thinking about this professional career option after getting licensed. It can be a very autonomous and rewarding experience; you just have to put the time and energy into it. This chapter was informed by some excellent resources with full citations provided in the References section below (Aronoff, 2017; Baumgarten, 2017; DaSilva, 2018; Grodzki, 2015). If you are still interested in private practice, it is never too early to start researching (and dreaming). Check out the sources cited here, but also take the time to find additional literature and peruse reputable websites as well. There is much to learn about private practice, but you will want to develop your own unique approach.

REFERENCES

Aronoff, K. (2017). *Best practice: Everything you need to know about starting your successful private therapy practice.* Author.

Baumgarten, H. (2017). *Private practice essentials: Business tools for mental health professionals.* PESI Publishing.

DaSilva, M. (2018). *The profitable private practice: How to start, run, and grow a therapy practice.* Author.

Grodzki, L. (2015). *Building your ideal private practice: A guide for therapists and other healing professionals* (2nd ed.). Norton & Company.

ADDITIONAL RESOURCES

Barnett, J. E., & Zimmerman, J. (2019). *If you build it they will come: And other myths of private practice in the mental health professions.* Oxford University Press.

Barnett, J. E., Zimmerman, J., & Walfish, S. (2017). *The ethics of private practice: A practical guide for mental health clinician.* Oxford University Press.

Bartolucci, A. D. (2017). *Business basics for private practice: A guide for mental health professionals.* Routledge.

Duan, M. L. (2019). *Starting your private practice: A step-by-step guide for mental health counselors.* Author.

Dwyer, K. (2020). *Intentional private practice workbook.* Author.

Olloh, C. N. (2021). *How to open a private practice mental health clinic within thirty days and marketing tips.* Author.

Waldman, L. (2021). *The graduate course you never had: How to develop, manage and market a flourishing private mental health practice* (2nd ed.). Outskirts Press.

Walfish, S., Barnett, J. E., & Zimmerman J. (2017). *Handbook of private practice: Keys to success for mental health practitioners.* Oxford University Press.

Wendler, D. (2016). *Clicking with clients: Online marketing for private practice therapists.* Author.

Appendix

State Key Requirements for Licensure

■ ■ ■

State	License Title/Name	Graduate Program Credit Hours	Graduate Program CACREP Accreditation Required?	Graduate Program Counseling Hours	Postgraduate Counseling Hours	Exam Required
Alabama http://www.abec.state.al.us/	Licensed Professional Counselor (LPC) Associate Licensed Counselor (ALC) A person licensed to render professional counseling services in private practice for a fee while under board supervision.	48	No	700 Total – 280 Direct and 2.5 hours per week supervised.	3,000 Total – including 2,250 hours of direct counseling services.	NCE

State	License Title/Name	Graduate Program Credit Hours	Graduate Program CACREP Accreditation Required?	Graduate Program Counseling Hours	Postgraduate Counseling Hours	Exam Required
Alaska https://www.commerce.alaska.gov/web/cbpl/Professional Licensing/Professional Counselors.aspx	Licensed Professional Counselor (LPC)	60	No	Not specified	3,000 Total – including 1,000 hours of direct counseling services and 100 hours of supervision.	NCE, NCMHCE, or successful completion of another nationally recognized examination for professional counselors that is equivalent to the NCE and/or NCMHCE.

State	License Title/Name	Graduate Program Credit Hours	Graduate Program CACREP Accreditation Required?	Graduate Program Counseling Hours	Postgraduate Counseling Hours	Exam Required
Arizona https://www.azbbhe.us/node/837	Licensed Professional Counselor (LPC) Licensed Associate Counselor (LAC) LAC's may only practice under direct supervision and shall not engage in independent practice.	60	Yes (or state board-approved program)	700 Total – including 240 hours of direct counseling.	3,200 Total – including 1,600 hours of direct counseling services and 100 hours of supervision.	NCE, NCMHCE, or CRCE

State	License Title/Name	Graduate Program Credit Hours	Graduate Program CACREP Accreditation Required?	Graduate Program Counseling Hours	Postgraduate Counseling Hours	Exam Required
Arkansas https://abec.state solutions.us/	Licensed Professional Counselor (LPC) Licensed Associate Counselor (LAC) An applicant with less than 3 years of post-master's-level supervision experience.	60	No	Not specified	3,000 Total	NCE and oral exam

State	License Title/Name	Graduate Program Credit Hours	Graduate Program CACREP Accreditation Required?	Graduate Program Counseling Hours	Postgraduate Counseling Hours	Exam Required
California https://calpcc.org/licensure-requirements	Licensed Professional Clinical Counselor (LPCC) Professional Clinical Counselor Intern (PCCI) An unlicensed person who has completed the educational requirements and is registered with the board to complete the supervision requirements to be licensed as an LPCC.	60	No	280 Total – All 280 hours must be direct counseling.	3,000 Total – All hours supervised and including 1,750 direct client contact hours.	NCMHCE and California Law and Ethics Examination

State	License Title/Name	Graduate Program Credit Hours	Graduate Program CACREP Accreditation Required?	Graduate Program Counseling Hours	Postgraduate Counseling Hours	Exam Required
Colorado https://www.colorado.gov/pacific/dora/Professional_Counselor_Laws	Licensed Professional Counselor (LPC) Licensed Professional Counselor Candidate (LPCC) An applicant who has completed the education requirements and is under a licensed supervisor; valid for 4 years.	60	No	700 Total	2,000 Total – Including 100 hours of supervision.	NCE and Colorado Jurisprudence Exam

State	License Title/Name	Graduate Program Credit Hours	Graduate Program CACREP Accreditation Required?	Graduate Program Counseling Hours	Postgraduate Counseling Hours	Exam Required
Connecticut https://portal.ct.gov/DPH/Practitioner-Licensing--Investigations/Professional-Counselor/Professional-Counselor-Licensing	Licensed Professional Counselor (LPC)	60	No	Not specified	3,000 Total – Including 100 hours of supervision.	NCE or NCMHCE

State	License Title/Name	Graduate Program Credit Hours	Graduate Program CACREP Accreditation Required?	Graduate Program Counseling Hours	Postgraduate Counseling Hours	Exam Required
Delaware https://dpr. delaware. gov/boards/ profcounselors/ newlicense/	Licensed Professional Counselor of Mental Health (LPCMH) Licensed Associate Counselor of Mental Health (LACMH) An individual licensed for the purpose of gaining experience required for licensure as an LPCMH.	60	No	Not specified	3,200 Total – of which 1,600 must be an approved supervisor (state board determined).	NCE or NCMHCE

State	License Title/Name	Graduate Program Credit Hours	Graduate Program CACREP Accreditation Required?	Graduate Program Counseling Hours	Postgraduate Counseling Hours	Exam Required
District of Columbia https:// dchealth. dc.gov/ service/ professional- counseling- initial- license- application- package	Licensed Professional Counselor (LPC) Licensed Graduate Professional Counselor (LGPC) An individual licensed for the purpose of gaining experience required for licensure as an LPC.	60	No	700 Total	3,500 Total – Including 200 hours of supervision.	NCE *Will accept NCMHCE or CRCE if already taken in another jurisdiction.

State	License Title/Name	Graduate Program Credit Hours	Graduate Program CACREP Accreditation Required?	Graduate Program Counseling Hours	Postgraduate Counseling Hours	Exam Required
Florida https:// floridasmental health professions.gov/ licensing/ licensed- mental-health- counselor/	Licensed Mental Health Counselor (LMHC) Provisional Mental Health Counselor A person provisionally licensed to provide mental health counseling under supervision.	60	No	1,000 Total – Including 280 direct counseling hours.	1,500 Total – Including 100 hours of supervision.	NCMHCE

State	License Title/Name	Graduate Program Credit Hours	Graduate Program CACREP Accreditation Required?	Graduate Program Counseling Hours	Postgraduate Counseling Hours	Exam Required
Georgia http://sos. ga.gov/ index.php/ licensing/ plb/43	Licensed Professional Counselor (LPC) Provisional Mental Health Counselor A person provisionally licensed to provide mental health counseling under supervision.	Not specified	No	600 Total	2,400 Total – Including 120 hours of supervision.	NCE

State	License Title/Name	Graduate Program Credit Hours	Graduate Program CACREP Accreditation Required?	Graduate Program Counseling Hours	Postgraduate Counseling Hours	Exam Required
Hawaii http://cca. hawaii. gov/pvl/ programs/ mental/	Licensed Mental Health Counselor (LMHC)	48	No	6 semester hours and 300 client contact hours total	3,000 Total – Including 100 hours of supervision.	NCE

State	License Title/Name	Graduate Program Credit Hours	Graduate Program CACREP Accreditation Required?	Graduate Program Counseling Hours	Postgraduate Counseling Hours	Exam Required
Idaho https:// ibol.idaho. gov/IBOL/ BoardPage. aspx?Bureau =COU	Licensed Clinical Professional Counselor (LCPC) Licensed Professional Counselor (LPC) Registered Counselor Intern A counselor performing under supervision as a part of the supervised experience requirement.	60	No	6 semester hours of practicum	LCPC 2,000 Total – Including 1,000 hours of supervision. LPC 1,000 Total – including 400 hours of direct client contact.	LCPC NCMHCE LPC NCE

State	License Title/Name	Graduate Program Credit Hours	Graduate Program CACREP Accreditation Required?	Graduate Program Counseling Hours	Postgraduate Counseling Hours	Exam Required
Illinois https://www.idfpr.com/profs/ProfCounselor.asp	Licensed Clinical Professional Counselor (LCPC) For independent practice of clinical professional counseling in private practice. Licensed Professional Counselor (LPC) Authorizes the practice of professional counseling.	48	No	Not specified	3,360 Total – Including 1,920 hours of direct service to clients.	LCPC NCE and NCMHCE or ECCP or CRCE LPC NCE or CRCE

State	License Title/Name	Graduate Program Credit Hours	Graduate Program CACREP Accreditation Required?	Graduate Program Counseling Hours	Postgraduate Counseling Hours	Exam Required
Indiana https://www.in.gov/pla/2888.htm	Licensed Mental Health Counselor (LMHC) Licensed Mental Health Counselor Associate (LMHCA) A counselor performing under the supervision as a part of the supervised experience requirement.	60	No	1,000 Total – Including 100 hours of supervision.	3,000 Total – Including 100 hours of supervision.	NCMHCE

State	License Title/Name	Graduate Program Credit Hours	Graduate Program CACREP Accreditation Required?	Graduate Program Counseling Hours	Postgraduate Counseling Hours	Exam Required
Iowa https://idph.iowa.gov/licensure/iowa-board-of-behavioral-science/licensure	Licensed Mental Health Counselor (LMHC) Temporary Licensed Mental Health Counselor (T-LMHC)	60	No	700 Total – Including 280 direct counseling hours and group therapy experience.	3,000 Total – Including 1,500 hours of direct client contact and 200 hours of supervision.	NCE or NCMHCE

State	License Title/Name	Graduate Program Credit Hours	Graduate Program CACREP Accreditation Required?	Graduate Program Counseling Hours	Postgraduate Counseling Hours	Exam Required
Kansas https://ksbsrb.ks.gov/professions/professional-counselors	Licensed Clinical Professional Counselor (LCPC) May diagnose and treat mental disorders independently. Licensed Professional Counselor (LPC) May practice under an LCPC.	60	No	350 Total – All 350 hours to be direct client contact.	4,000 Total – Including 1,500 hours of direct client contact and 150 hours of supervision.	NCE

State	License Title/Name	Graduate Program Credit Hours	Graduate Program CACREP Accreditation Required?	Graduate Program Counseling Hours	Postgraduate Counseling Hours	Exam Required
Kentucky https://lpc.ky.gov/	Licensed Professional Clinical Counselor (LPCC) Licensed Professional Counselor Associate (LPCA) An individual who has met all qualifications to engage in the practice of professional counseling under an approved clinical supervisor authorized by the board.	60	Yes	400 Total	4,000 Total – Including 1,600 hours of direct client contact and 100 hours of supervision.	NCE

State	License Title/Name	Graduate Program Credit Hours	Graduate Program CACREP Accreditation Required?	Graduate Program Counseling Hours	Postgraduate Counseling Hours	Exam Required
Louisiana http://www.lpcboard.org/	Licensed Professional Counselor (LPC) Provisional Licensed Professional Counselor (P-LPC) Individuals with a master's degree in counseling with practicing counseling under the board-approved supervision of an LPC.	60	No	400 Total – Including 160 hours of supervision.	3,000 Total – Including 1,900 direct client contact experience, 1,000 indirect client contact hours, and 100 face-to-face supervision hours	NCE or NCMHCE

State	License Title/Name	Graduate Program Credit Hours	Graduate Program CACREP Accreditation Required?	Graduate Program Counseling Hours	Postgraduate Counseling Hours	Exam Required
Maine https://www.maine.gov/pfr/professional licensing/professions/counselors/index.html	Licensed Clinical Professional Counselor (LCPC) Licensed Professional Counselor (LPC) Conditional LCPC A license granted to an applicant for licensure as an LCPC who has met all the requirements except for the supervised clinical experience. Conditional LPC A license granted to an applicant for licensure as an LPC who has met all the requirements except for the supervised clinical experience.	LCPC 60 LPC 48	No	LCPC 1,000 Total – Including 400 hours of direct client contact. LPC 700 Total – Including 280 hours of direct client contact.	LCPC 3,000 Total – Including 1,500 hours of direct client contact and 1 hour of clinical supervision per 30 hours of client contact. LPC 2,000 total – Including 1,000 hours of direct counseling and 67 hours of supervision.	LCPC NCMHCE LPC NCE

State	License Title/Name	Graduate Program Credit Hours	Graduate Program CACREP Accreditation Required?	Graduate Program Counseling Hours	Postgraduate Counseling Hours	Exam Required
Maryland https://health.maryland.gov/bopc/Pages/pc.aspx	Licensed Clinical Professional Counselor (LCPC) Licensed Graduate Professional Counselor (LGPC) Title used while fulfilling the supervised clinical experience requirement.	60	No	1,000 Total	2,000 Total – Including 100 hours of supervision.	NCE and Maryland Professional Counselors and Therapists Act Exam.

State	License Title/Name	Graduate Program Credit Hours	Graduate Program CACREP Accreditation Required?	Graduate Program Counseling Hours	Postgraduate Counseling Hours	Exam Required
Massachusetts https://www.mass.gov/lists/statutes-and-regulations-allied-mental-health	Licensed Mental Health Counselor (LMHC)	60	No	700 Total – Including 280 hours of direct client counseling hours and 70 hours of supervision in a practicum and an internship.	3,360 Total – Including 960 hours of direct client contact and 130 hours of supervision.	NCMHCE

State	License Title/Name	Graduate Program Credit Hours	Graduate Program CACREP Accreditation Required?	Graduate Program Counseling Hours	Postgraduate Counseling Hours	Exam Required
Michigan https://www. michigan.gov/ lara/0,4601,7-154-72600_ 72603_27529_ 27536---,00. html	Licensed Professional Counselor (LPC) Limited Licensed Professional Counselor (LLPC) A limited license is issued to those who have not yet completed the 3,000-hour supervised counseling experience.	48	No	600 hours internship	3,000 Total – Including 100 hours of supervision.	NCE or CRCE

State	License Title/Name	Graduate Program Credit Hours	Graduate Program CACREP Accreditation Required?	Graduate Program Counseling Hours	Postgraduate Counseling Hours	Exam Required
Minnesota https:// mn.gov/ boards/ behavioral-health/ statutes-and-rules/lpc-lpcc-statutes-rules/ lpc-lpcc-statutes.jsp	Licensed Professional Clinical Counselor (LPCC) Licensed Professional Counselor (LPC)	48	No	700 Total	LPCC 4,000 Total – Including 1,800 direct client hours. LPC 2,000 Total	LPCC NCMHCE LPC NCE or other national exam that is determined by the board to be substantially similar to the NCE.

State	License Title/Name	Graduate Program Credit Hours	Graduate Program CACREP Accreditation Required?	Graduate Program Counseling Hours	Postgraduate Counseling Hours	Exam Required
Mississippi https://www.lpc.ms.gov/secure/index.asp	Licensed Professional Counselor (LPC) Provisional Licensed Professional Counselor (P-LPC) Applicant who has completed master's degree and has completed NCE, but requires supervision to meet counseling requirements satisfied.	60	No	Up to 1,750 hours can be obtained	3,500 Total – Including 1,167 hours of direct client contact and 100 hours of supervision.	NCMHCE

State	License Title/Name	Graduate Program Credit Hours	Graduate Program CACREP Accreditation Required?	Graduate Program Counseling Hours	Postgraduate Counseling Hours	Exam Required
Missouri https://pr.mo.gov/counselors.asp	Licensed Professional Counselor (LPC) Counselor-in-Training Issued automatically when supervision is registered and approved and all other requirements are met.	48	No (If an online program, must be mental health counseling and CACREP accredited)	Not specified	3,000 Total – Including 1,200 hours of direct client contact and 15 hours of supervision per week.	NCE and Missouri Jurisprudence Exam

State	License Title/Name	Graduate Program Credit Hours	Graduate Program CACREP Accreditation Required?	Graduate Program Counseling Hours	Postgraduate Counseling Hours	Exam Required
Montana http://boards.bsd.dli.mt.gov/bbh#1	Licensed Clinical Professional Counselor (LCPC)	60	No	Up to 1,500 hours can be obtained	3,000 Total – Including pre-master's hours, 1,000 hours of direct client contact, and 1 hour of supervision for every 20 hours.	NCE and NCMHCE

State	License Title/Name	Graduate Program Credit Hours	Graduate Program CACREP Accreditation Required?	Graduate Program Counseling Hours	Postgraduate Counseling Hours	Exam Required
Nebraska http://dhhs.ne.gov/licensure/Pages/Mental-Health-and-Social-Work-Practice.aspx	Licensed Mental Health Practitioner (LCPC) An individual who is qualified to engage in mental health practice or offers or renders mental health practice services. Provisionally Licensed Mental Health Practitioner (PLMHP) An individual earning experience toward the LMHP/LIMPH.	Not specified	No	300 Total	3,000 Total – Including pre-master's hours, 1,500 hours of direct client contact.	NCE or NCMHCE

State	License Title/Name	Graduate Program Credit Hours	Graduate Program CACREP Accreditation Required?	Graduate Program Counseling Hours	Postgraduate Counseling Hours	Exam Required
Nevada http://marriage.nv.gov/Services/CPC/	Clinical Professional Counselor (CPC) Licensed Clinical Professional Counselor Intern Required before beginning supervised experience after obtaining valid master's degree.	48	No	Not specified	3,000 Total – Including pre-master's hours, 1,500 hours of direct client contact, and 300 hours of supervision.	NCMHCE

State	License Title/Name	Graduate Program Credit Hours	Graduate Program CACREP Accreditation Required?	Graduate Program Counseling Hours	Postgraduate Counseling Hours	Exam Required
New Hampshire https://www.oplc.nh.gov/mental-health/	Licensed Clinical Mental Health Counselor (LCMHC)	60	No	700 Total	3,000 Total – Including 100 hours of supervision.	NCMHCE

State	License Title/Name	Graduate Program Credit Hours	Graduate Program CACREP Accreditation Required?	Graduate Program Counseling Hours	Postgraduate Counseling Hours	Exam Required
New Jersey https://www. njconsumer affairs.gov/ pc/Pages/ default.aspx	Licensed Clinical Mental Health Counselor (LCMHC) An LPC can apply for this specialty designation after satisfying the continuing education requirements of the committee. Licensed Professional Counselor (LPC) Associate Licensed Counselor (ALC) After acceptable documentation of satisfaction of the LPC educational and examination requirements, an individual may be granted licensure as an Associate Counselor to practice counseling under direct supervision.	60	No	Up to 1,500 hours can be obtained.	3,000 Total – Including pre-master's hours and 100 hours of face-to-face supervision. LPC 3 years of full-time supervised counseling experience, 1 year of which can be obtained prior to the granting of the master's degree.	NCE

State	License Title/Name	Graduate Program Credit Hours	Graduate Program CACREP Accreditation Required?	Graduate Program Counseling Hours	Postgraduate Counseling Hours	Exam Required
New Mexico http://www.rld.state.nm.us/boards/counseling_and_therapy_practice_forms_and_applications.aspx	Licensed Professional Clinical Mental Health Counselor (LPCC) Licensed Mental Health Counselor (LMHC) Individuals who are pursuing the LPCC license but still need to complete the supervised experience requirements.	48	No	Up to 1,000 hours can be obtained.	3,000 Total – Including pre-master's hours and 100 hours of supervision.	LPCC NCE and NCMHCE LMHC NCE

State	License Title/Name	Graduate Program Credit Hours	Graduate Program CACREP Accreditation Required?	Graduate Program Counseling Hours	Postgraduate Counseling Hours	Exam Required
New York http://www.op.nysed.gov/prof/mhp/mhclic.htm	Licensed Mental Health Counselor (LMHC) Limited Permit Applicants who have met all requirements except experience and/or exam must apply for a 2-year permit to practice under supervision.	60	No	600 Total	3,000 Total – Including 1,500 hours of direct client contact and 4 hours per month of supervision.	NCMHCE

State	License Title/Name	Graduate Program Credit Hours	Graduate Program CACREP Accreditation Required?	Graduate Program Counseling Hours	Postgraduate Counseling Hours	Exam Required
North Carolina http://www.ncblpc.org/	Licensed Clinical Mental Health Counselor (LCMHC) Licensed Clinical Mental Health Counselor Associate (LCMHCA) Individuals who are pursuing the LCMHC license but still need to complete the supervised professional practice experience requirements.	60	Yes	300 Total – Including 180 direct client hours.	3,000 Total – Including 2,000 hours of direct client contact and 100 hours of supervision.	NCE, NCMHCE, or CRCE and North Carolina Jurisprudence Exam.

State	License Title/Name	Graduate Program Credit Hours	Graduate Program CACREP Accreditation Required?	Graduate Program Counseling Hours	Postgraduate Counseling Hours	Exam Required
North Dakota http://www.ndbce.org/LPCC.shtml	Licensed Professional Clinical Counselor (LPCC) Advanced license. Licensed Professional Counselor (LPC) Full professional license. Licensed Associate Professional Counselor (LAPC) A two-year license that allows the completion of the supervised experience.	60	No	700 Total	LPCC 3,000 Total – Including 100 hours of supervision. LPC 400 – direct client counseling.	LPCC NCMHCE and a videotaped clinical counseling session of at least 30 minutes. LPC/LAPC NCE

State	License Title/Name	Graduate Program Credit Hours	Graduate Program CACREP Accreditation Required?	Graduate Program Counseling Hours	Postgraduate Counseling Hours	Exam Required
Ohio https:// cswmft. ohio. gov/wps/ portal/gov/ cswmft/get-licensed/ counselors	**Licensed Professional Clinical Counselor (LPCC)** **Professional Counselor/ Clinical Resident** (CR) Title used while completing the 3,000 hours of supervised experience required for the LPCC license. **Licensed Professional Counselor (LPC)** Title used after completing coursework including practicum and internship. **Registered Counselor Trainee** (RCT) Title used while enrolled in a practicum or internship in a counselor education program.	60	No	700 Total – Including 100-hour practicum and 600-hour internship.	3,000 Total – Including 150 hours of supervision.	NCMHCE, NCE, and Ohio Jurisprudence Exam

State	License Title/Name	Graduate Program Credit Hours	Graduate Program CACREP Accreditation Required?	Graduate Program Counseling Hours	Postgraduate Counseling Hours	Exam Required
Oklahoma https://www.ok.gov/behavioral health/	Licensed Professional Counselor (LPC) Licensed Professional Counselor Candidate (LPC-candidate) An individual may be granted licensure as a Licensed Professional Counselor Candidate to practice counseling under the direct supervision of an approved LPC supervisor.	60	No	300 Total	3,000 Total	NCE and Oklahoma Legal and Ethical Responsibilities Exam

State	License Title/Name	Graduate Program Credit Hours	Graduate Program CACREP Accreditation Required?	Graduate Program Counseling Hours	Postgraduate Counseling Hours	Exam Required
Oregon https://www.oregon.gov/oblpct/Pages/index.aspx	Licensed Professional Counselor (LPC) Registered Intern An applicant registered to obtain post-degree supervised work experience toward licensure.	60	No	700 Total – Including 280 direct client counseling hours.	2,400 Total – direct client contact.	NCE, NCMHCE, CRCE, or other exam, as approved by the board; and Oregon Law and Rules Exam

State	License Title/Name	Graduate Program Credit Hours	Graduate Program CACREP Accreditation Required?	Graduate Program Counseling Hours	Postgraduate Counseling Hours	Exam Required
Pennsylvania https://www.dos.pa.gov/Professional Licensing/Boards Commissions/SocialWorkers Marriagean FamilyTherapists andProfessional Counselors/Pages/Board-Laws-and-Regulations.aspx#.VG-alVZOk5s	Licensed Professional Counselor (LPC)	60	No	700 Total – Including 100-hour practicum and 600-hour internship.	3,000 Total – Including 150 hours of supervision.	NCE or CRCE

State (Territory)	License Title/Name	Graduate Program Credit Hours	Graduate Program CACREP Accreditation Required?	Graduate Program Counseling Hours	Postgraduate Counseling Hours	Exam Required
Puerto Rico www.salud. gov.pr	Licensed Professional Counselor (LPC) Professional Counselor with Provisional License (PCPL) A person who is granted a temporary/ provisional authorization by the board to offer counseling services under the supervision to meet the experience requirement.	45	No	Not specified	500 Total	NCE

State	License Title/Name	Graduate Program Credit Hours	Graduate Program CACREP Accreditation Required?	Graduate Program Counseling Hours	Postgraduate Counseling Hours	Exam Required
Rhode Island http:// health. ri.gov/ licenses/ detail. php?id=228	Mental Health Counselor (MHC)	60	No	Internship of 20 counseling per week for one calendar year.	2,000 Total – Including 100 hours of supervision.	NCMHCE

State	License Title/Name	Graduate Program Credit Hours	Graduate Program CACREP Accreditation Required?	Graduate Program Counseling Hours	Postgraduate Counseling Hours	Exam Required
South Carolina https://www.llr.sc.gov/pol/counselors/index.asp?file=pub.htm	Licensed Professional Counselor (LPC) Licensed Professional Counselor Associate (LPC/A) An applicant who has met the education and exam requirements but not the 2 years' supervised experience requirement.	60	No	700 Total	1,500 Total – including 150 hours of supervision.	NCE or NCMHCE

State	License Title/Name	Graduate Program Credit Hours	Graduate Program CACREP Accreditation Required?	Graduate Program Counseling Hours	Postgraduate Counseling Hours	Exam Required
South Dakota https://dss.sd.gov/licensing boards/counselors/counselors.aspx	Licensed Professional Counselor – Mental Health (LPC-MH) Licensed Professional Counselor (LPC)	LPC-MH 48 LPC 48	No	700 Total – Including 100-hour practicum and 600-hour internship.	LPC-MH 2,000 Total – direct client contact total, including hours earned under the LPC License and 100 hours of supervision. LPC 2,000 Total – counseling experience, including 800 hours of direct client contact	LPC-MH NCMHCE LPC NCE

State	License Title/Name	Graduate Program Credit Hours	Graduate Program CACREP Accreditation Required?	Graduate Program Counseling Hours	Postgraduate Counseling Hours	Exam Required
Tennessee https://www.tn.gov/health/health-program-areas/health-professional-boards/pcmft-board/pcmft-board/licensure.html	Licensed Professional Counselor – Mental Health Service Provider (LPC/MHSP) Individuals with the LPC/MHSP licensure can assess and diagnose under the DSM-5. Licensed Professional Counselor (LPC)	60	No	500 Total	LPC/MHSP 3,000 Total – including 1,500 direct client contact hours, 1,500 clinically based hours, and 150 hours of supervision. LPC 2,100 total – including 2,000 direct client contact hours and 100 hours of supervision.	LPC-MH NCE, NCMHCE, and the Tennessee Jurisprudence Exam LPC NCE and the Tennessee Jurisprudence Exam

State	License Title/Name	Graduate Program Credit Hours	Graduate Program CACREP Accreditation Required?	Graduate Program Counseling Hours	Postgraduate Counseling Hours	Exam Required
Texas https://dshs.texas.gov/counselor/	Licensed Professional Counselor (LPC) Licensed Professional Counselor Intern (LPC-I) An applicant practicing under supervision.	60	No	300 Total – Including 100 hours of direct client contact.	3,000 Total – Including 1,500 hours of direct client contact.	NCE or NCMHCE and Texas Jurisprudence Exam.

State	License Title/Name	Graduate Program Credit Hours	Graduate Program CACREP Accreditation Required?	Graduate Program Counseling Hours	Postgraduate Counseling Hours	Exam Required
Utah https:// dopl.utah. gov/cmhc/ index. html	Clinical Mental Health Counselor (CMHC) Associate Clinical Mental Health Counselor (ACMHC) License required before starting the supervised experience requirement.	60	No	1,000 Total – Including 400 hours of direct client contact.	4,000 Total – Including 100 hours of supervision	NCE and NCMHCE

State	License Title/Name	Graduate Program Credit Hours	Graduate Program CACREP Accreditation Required?	Graduate Program Counseling Hours	Postgraduate Counseling Hours	Exam Required
Vermont https://sos. vermont. gov/allied-mental-health/ forms-instructions/	Licensed Clinical Mental Health Counselor (LCMHC)	60	No	700 Total	3,000 Total – Including 2,000 hours of direct client contact and 100 hours of supervision.	NCE, NCMHCE, and Vermont Jurisprudence Exam.

State	License Title/Name	Graduate Program Credit Hours	Graduate Program CACREP Accreditation Required?	Graduate Program Counseling Hours	Postgraduate Counseling Hours	Exam Required
Virginia https://www.dhp.virginia.gov/counseling/counseling_forms.htm#LPC	Licensed Professional Counselor (LPC) Licensed Professional Counselor – Resident (LPC-Resident) An applicant practicing under supervision.	60	No	600 Total – Including 240 hours of direct client contact.	3,400 Total – Including 2,000 hours of direct client contact and 200 hours of supervision.	NCMHCE

State	License Title/Name	Graduate Program Credit Hours	Graduate Program CACREP Accreditation Required?	Graduate Program Counseling Hours	Postgraduate Counseling Hours	Exam Required
Washington https://www.doh.wa.gov/LicensesPermitsand Certificates/ProfessionsNew ReneworUpdate/Mental Health Counselor	Licensed Mental Health Counselor (LMHC) Licensed Mental Health Counselor Associate (LMHCA) A candidate who has a graduate degree in mental health counseling or related field and is working toward meeting the supervised experience requirements.	60	No	Not specified	3,000 Total – Including 1,200 hours of direct client contact and 100 hours of supervision.	NCE or NCMHCE

State	License Title/Name	Graduate Program Credit Hours	Graduate Program CACREP Accreditation Required?	Graduate Program Counseling Hours	Postgraduate Counseling Hours	Exam Required
West Virginia http://www.wvbec.org/	Licensed Professional Counselor (LPC) Licensed Mental Health Counselor Associate (LMHCA) A candidate who has a graduate degree in mental health counseling or related field and is working toward meeting the supervised experience requirements.	60	No	Up to 600 – Can be counted toward 3,000 total required.	3,000 Total – Including 1,500 hours of direct client contact.	NCE, CRCE, or NCMHCE

State	License Title/Name	Graduate Program Credit Hours	Graduate Program CACREP Accreditation Required?	Graduate Program Counseling Hours	Postgraduate Counseling Hours	Exam Required
Wisconsin https://dsps.wi.gov/Pages/Professions/LPC/Default.aspx	Licensed Professional Counselor (LPC) Licensed Professional Counselor Trainee An applicant who has completed the degree requirements but not the supervised experience.	60	No	Not specified	3,000 Total – Including 1,000 hours of direct client contact.	NCE, CRCE, or NCMHCE Wisconsin Jurisprudence Exam (for reciprocity applicants only)

State	License Title/Name	Graduate Program Credit Hours	Graduate Program CACREP Accreditation Required?	Graduate Program Counseling Hours	Postgraduate Counseling Hours	Exam Required
Wyoming http:// mentalhealth. wyo.gov/	Licensed Professional Counselor (LPC) Provisional Professional Counselor (PPC) An applicant who has received a master's degree but has not passed the exam or completed the supervised experience requirement.	60	No	700 Total – 100 practicum hours and 600 internship hours, 240 of which are direct client contact	3,000 Total – Including 1,200 hours of direct client contact and 100 hours of supervision.	NCE, CRCE, or NCMHCE

Index

■ ■ ■

About the Author

■ ■ ■

Adam M. Volungis, Ph.D. is a counseling psychologist and licensed mental health counselor. He has worked with a variety of populations in multiple settings using CBT for the past 15+ years. Dr. Volungis is an associate professor and the cognitive-behavioral therapies concentration coordinator in the Clinical Counseling Psychology Program (CCPP) at Assumption University (Worcester, MA) where he teaches multiple CBT graduate courses. The CCPP is home to the Aaron T. Beck Institute for Cognitive Studies and is one of the few master's-level programs in the country with a primary concentration in cognitive-behavioral studies. He is a member of the American Mental Health Counselors Association, American Psychological Association, Association for Behavioral and Cognitive Therapies, Eastern Psychological Association, and New England Psychological Association. He is also president of the New England Psychological Association (2021–2023) and the author of *Cognitive-Behavioral Therapy: Theory into Practice* (published by Rowman & Littlefield).

www.ingramcontent.com/pod-product-compliance
Lightning Source LLC
Chambersburg PA
CBHW060154280326
41932CB00012B/1755